THE
7 O'CLOCK
BEDTIME

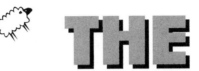

THE
7 O'CLOCK
BEDTIME

Inda Schaenen

ReganBooks
An Imprint of HarperCollins*Publishers*

HarperCollins books may be purchased for educational, business, or sales promotional use. For information please write: Special Markets Department, HarperCollins Publishers Inc., 10 East 53rd Street, New York, NY 10022.

FIRST EDITION

Designed by Jessica Shatan

Library of Congress Cataloging-in-Publication Data

Schaenen, Inda.
  The 7 o'clock bedtime / Inda Schaenen.
    p. cm.
  Includes bibliographical references and index.
  ISBN 0-06-098889-4
  1. Sleep disorders in children—Popular works. 2. Children—Sleep—Popular works. I. Title: 7 o'clock bedtime. II. Title.

RJ506.S55 S345 2001
618.92'8498—dc21   00-067356

01 02 03 04 05 RRD 10 9 8 7 6 5 4 3 2 1

To my husband and
our children

Only that day dawns to which we are awake.

—HENRY DAVID THOREAU, *Walden*

Contents

Foreword

The 7 o'clock bedtime . . . to a weary, bleary-eyed veteran of the daily skirmishes of parenthood, the phrase is like a clarion call. It conjures up myriad fantasies: evenings spent in glorious solitude, romantic spousal reacquainting dinners, hour-long bubble bath marathons, a pottery class here, a *New York Times* bestseller read in one sitting there. It has the power to evoke heady visions of Dr. Denton pajama–clad, apple-cheeked moppets marching cheerily off to dreamland, only to wake the following morning with well-scrubbed and smiling faces to greet the new day. . . .

What interrupts, of course, with boorish swiftness, are the voices of Reason, Doubt, and Guilt, those constant comrades-in-arms of the working parent. What about cutting into Quality Time, we protest, a transgression second only to a diet consisting solely of french fries in the modern parent's handbook of deadly sins? What child, we sigh, when faced with the lure of the Cartoon Network or the seductive glow of a flickering computer screen, would actually choose bed? (At least without a protest, the magnitude of which defies both imagination and our already

meager coping strategies?) And besides, we reason, isn't it cruel?
So, reluctantly, we place this slim volume back on the bookstore
shelf for some other better, stronger, wiser parent to pick up and
employ.

Don't. I am here to tell you that you are that better, stronger,
wiser parent, whether you believe it or not. And what will make
that possible, as so eloquently argued by Inda Schaenen, will be
your newfound, unswerving, well-reasoned conviction that this is
in the best interest of your child. Once persuaded that a good
night's sleep, much like nutrition, seat belts, and a roof over one's
head, is not only an inalienable right of every child and parent
but a bona fide parental responsibility, you are more than halfway
there.

And if Ms. Schaenen's elegant prose is not quite enough to
convince you, heed this. There is a growing body of scientific
literature, certain to expand significantly in the next few years,
that demonstrates clearly the often dire consequences of inade-
quate sleep in children, ranging from mood disturbances (what
we behavioral scientists like to term *lack of positive affect*, and
what every parent recognizes as *the crankies*), to deficits in
attention and short-term memory, to poor performance in the
classroom. Coupled with these empirical arguments is the clinical experience of a host of pediatric professionals like me, who
have directly observed over and over again in our small, sleep-
deprived patients the link between poor sleep and behavior
problems, school failure, and attention deficit hyperactivity disorder. Not to mention the teachers, school nurses, guidance counselors, and coaches who must struggle daily with the aftermath of
what I have come to call (with apologies to the folks at Disney)
the *Sleepy, Dopey, Grumpy Syndrome*.

So take heart. If the old adage "you reap what you sow" con-
tains even a grain of truth, you and your child will reap the benefits of the sandman's sack a thousandfold. And while you're at it,

you might just find that *you* don't need that second double-shot espresso mocha latte to have a good day.

—Judith A. Owens, M.D., M.P.H., director, Pediatric Sleep Disorders Clinic; director, Learning, Attention, and Behavior Program, Hasbro Children's Hospital; associate professor of pediatrics, Brown University School of Medicine

THE
7 O'CLOCK
BEDTIME

Introduction

It's ten past seven on a Monday night. I am the only adult in the house (my husband is working late), and I've just put our three children—ages ten, seven, and four—to bed. I promise you this is true. What's more, with the exceptions resulting from special events, illness, and travel, it's true almost every single night of the week: seven o'clock means bedtime.

Most people laugh at me. Some envy me. Some scorn my adherence to an apparently draconian schedule, call me a rigid control freak. What can I say? Call me anything you want, just don't call me after seven at night, because that's when I am totally off duty, at least as a mother. My parenting day done, I have a few hours every evening to use as I wish. When the children were very young and I had no free time during the day, I used to leave my husband home with them and pop out two or three times a week for a seven-thirty aerobics class. These days, I usually head for my desk and perform the work I actually get paid to do. Other nights I crawl into bed at seven-fifteen, read for an hour, and spend the next ten hours catching up on my own sleep. Some evenings I spend with my husband, either at home or out for dinner and a movie.

But whatever I do, the evening hours are my own, and my children get enough sleep to grow on.

If you are completely happy with the rhythms of your family life, feel free to stop reading right now. But if something feels wrong about your days and nights; if your kids are harried, cranky, and unpleasant; if they are having trouble in school or their behavior is not up to your standards or expectations; if you end each day angry and resentful, or guilty and fretful; or if it seems to you that your children have more say in their bedtime than you do, then you may well think about how you might manage things differently.

Naturally, it is much easier to set up a routine when your first baby is very young. But if you are convinced that having an early routine is a good thing for you, I am sure it is possible to help even older children make the changes you need to make. While I may refer from time to time to the needs of teenagers, I am confining this book to the years between infancy and the onset of puberty. How teenage biology relates to teenage sleep is a lively field unto itself, a field currently being studied by researchers like Mary Carskadon at Brown University, Carla Wahlstrom at the University of Minnesota, and many others. Physical and chemical changes in the teenager's brain lend themselves to multiple interpretations. In addition to biology, other variables such as part-time jobs, onerous loads of homework, after-school activities, increased social independence, and school starting times factor into the sleep of adolescents. Their habits and routines are beyond the scope of this book.

It's hard not to wonder, though, whether the patterns we have established during their prepubescent years will sustain our children as they grow into teenagers. I have no idea. I doubt that three years from now my ten-year-old will be closing her eyes at seven-thirty; I can, however, imagine that because of her childhood rhythms, she may be more likely to remain the early bird she has always been. Certainly, because she is being raised to respect her biological need for an adequate amount of sleep, she will assume that regulating her hours of sleep is as important as regulating her consumption of cookies after a meal.

Please understand, then, that the very concept of the 7 o'clock bedtime can be understood metaphorically, as representative of a larger set of values parents may wish to impart to their children regarding the rhythm of daily life. If you accept that the most significant organizing principle and determining factor in a child's day is his sleep, then you will be more comfortable considering the adjustments and sacrifices this principle demands. Establishing an early bedtime is a highly personal and individual choice, one that requires you to see the big picture at all times. It helps if you conceive of enforced, obligatory wakefulness as shocking as the idea of tying children to mattresses and gluing their eyelids shut.

●   ●   ●

"It is just as important to help our children maintain consistent schedules through infancy, childhood, and adolescence," Richard Ferber writes in his canonical if controversial book *Solve Your Child's Sleep Problems*. "In fact all of us, regardless of age, function best when we keep regular schedules. Studies in adults have shown that irregular sleep-wake patterns lead to significant alterations in our moods and sense of well-being, and undermine our ability to sleep at the desired times. The same is true of young children, although many parents don't seem to appreciate this fact."

It took me some time before I was ready to straighten out the sleep of our first child. Throughout her infancy she awoke several times throughout the night. At the time, I didn't even classify this as a problem. Babies are designed to rouse in the night, I told myself. They need the comfort and feel of their mother, I told myself. Midnight suckling and family beds are natural, I told myself. After fourteen months of utterly wrecked sleep, however, I began to tell myself a few other things. By then I wanted it both ways: the warmth and intimacy of a family bed, and a baby who slept through the night. A challenge, to say the least. And even though we managed to work these things out over time, our daughter continued to wake up every morning much, much earlier than we liked. No matter what time we put her to bed, she greeted the day around five-thirty or six the next morning. She was (and remains) what sleep specialists call an extreme lark. Given this kind of child, it behooved us to find a rhythm that helped her log in the hours asleep that she required as she grew.

By the time her brother was born she was two and a half years old. She napped from eleven-thirty to one-thirty, sometimes longer, and went to bed at seven o'clock. Fully expecting to alter the routine as her brother matured, I was instead surprised over the years by how bedtime stuck. When our third child was born, the early bedtime was so ingrained in all of us that we saw no reason to change anything. Partly because of his place in the family and partly because of his constitution, our youngest seems to have the greatest natural stamina of the three. Keeping up is his way of life. Nevertheless, he neither balks nor complains at bedtime, even when he's not as desperate for bed as his siblings.

In spite of having the same official bedtime, each of our children approaches the actual moment of falling asleep with his own individual personality and unique set of needs. There are children who need to babble and chat to themselves before falling asleep. There are children who seem to fall asleep the moment their eyes close. There are children who need to lie quietly, thinking, before shutting down for the day. Throughout their lives, my children have each fallen into each of these categories at one time or another. A physically exhausting day may knock out a four-year-old like a blow to the head; the same kind of day may rev up the mind of a nine-year-old. It helps to consider bedtime—firm and nonnegotiable as a starting line—as the night's beginning rather than as the day's end.

You need to know this too before we go any further: I still have firsthand experience with bedtimes from hell. As a matter of fact, I experienced such a moment last night with my older son. But here's the thing: his misery (caused by sleep deprivation from a late-arriving airplane after a fun-filled weekend out of town) lasted all of fifteen minutes. He and his weeping younger brother, whose tears were provoked by example, were in bed and falling asleep by six-thirty. That was it. Putting your children on an early schedule does not prevent monstrous endings to glorious days. It merely enables you to help your child out of his misery, the kind of misery that makes everyone in the family miserable. A child wears his fatigue like a suit of itchy, ill-fitting clothing. Putting him to bed with authority and affection may be likened to helping him out of the unbearably uncomfortable outfit and into a pair of well-worn pajamas.

I'm not going to tell you that you can create for yourself a perfect child, a perfect family, and a perfect bedtime. There are no such things. Nor should there be. Just as an all-sunny life would be an inhuman life, so a bedtime without a pang of regret at the loss of another day would be an inhuman bedtime. Bedtime can be loving, happy, peaceful, and sacred; but it always marks a bittersweet separation and an end. If you accept even this much, you will be that much more patient with your child's resistance to going to sleep.

Being patient, however, is not the same thing as being permissive.

The object of this book is to show you how to make bedtime firm and reliable, with just enough built-in flexibility to allow for life's vagaries. But as you'll see, bedtime doesn't begin at the end of the day. Bedtime is the denouement of each day's story. How you and your children write that story affects every aspect of bedtime.

● ● ●

I've drawn my conclusions from intellect, instinct, and experience; interviews with teachers, school administrators, day care directors, sleep specialists, child psychologists, and sleep researchers; the stories told by friends; and a layman's familiarity with child development literature. From the start, a few things seemed obvious to me:

- Once you have determined how much sleep your child needs, her need for that much sleep is nonnegotiable. Age-specific requirements will follow in chapter 1. Different kids require different amounts of sleep, and some may need as much as fourteen hours of sleep in every twenty-four-hour period.

- Children flourish when they are unhurried.

- Watching television is unnecessary.

- Playing computer games—even so-called educational games, both handheld and desktop—is unnecessary.

- Kids need time to play freely, outside if possible, every day.

- Prepubescent children do not need to busy themselves more than once a week after school with activities like karate, painting classes, modern jazz dancing, music lessons, and organized athletics.

- Parents are happiest when they know in advance what time their parenting day will end.

- Unconditional love for children is essential, but raising decent children also requires the consistent exercise of ingenuity, humor, intelligence, and self-discipline, all of which require an enormous amount of emotional and psychological stamina. In short, parents need sleep too.

There is nothing brilliantly insightful about the above list, nothing earth-shattering or newsy about it either, nor anything that ought to make anyone curse me for a raving ideologue. On the other hand, if you really take these premises to heart, if you live by them, then suddenly you find yourself making choices that place you in a minority that includes a wide variety of culture-bashing party poopers as well as those whom you consider your theoretical soul mates. Early bedtimes create curious bedfellows.

Further, the parenting arena is so emotionally supercharged and so easily dragged into the cockfighting pit of politics that I would be disingenuous to speak about 7 o'clock bedtimes without at least acknowledging that this plan works best for those in a position to care for children (or at least micromanage such care from afar) day in and day out. While nannies, baby-sitters, and extended family surrogates can step into any kind of routine, it seems entirely unreasonable to expect that children who are in day care or after-school programs until six will be fed and put to bed by seven o'clock. It probably could be accomplished, but who would want to? A parent who hasn't seen her child since eight in the morning is not likely to hasten home and toss the kid in bed within an hour. Nothing inherent in day care prevents early bedtimes (apart from allowing older preschoolers to nap when they would otherwise be growing out of the midday sleep; such a child is less likely to fall asleep early), and good centers all follow afternoon and early evening routines that resemble what I will be detailing below.

Of course, a parent picking up his child at six might reason that a cranky four-year-old might just as well be put to bed at seven o'clock and awaken fresh and ready for parental attention at five-thirty or six the next morning. Trading the harried evening hour for a quiet morning hour might be, for some, a viable alternative. Parents of long-sleepers may find that it's in their child's best interest to lose nearly all of the so-called quality time with the parent for the sake of the rest the child seems to need at that point in his development. But again, these scenarios represent extremely personal choices, choices that are made against a backdrop of day care facilities whose quality ranges across a broad spectrum from center to center, and of parental psychology which, almost by definition, incorporates a certain level of ambivalence.

It's too bad day care is not universally good. It's too bad male and female college graduates don't flock into the profession of day care the way they flock into banking, law, and business. If those who cared for kids appropriately and skillfully—the "allomothers" of both sexes—could be remunerated fairly for their skills, those who haven't a clue about (or an interest in) child development could pursue their own professions without wreaking havoc on the next generation—and with less guilt. But obviously, we're not there yet.

To be sure, child-rearing practices change within a culture as the culture itself evolves. As a rule, the most popular voices in the field (writers, journalists, and child experts) are those who praise practices that serve the current economy. Collectively they constitute The Voice, and The Voice is very hard to ignore. When, for example, women are engaged in the workforce in large numbers (as during World War II and now), The Voice touts collective all-day day care as particularly beneficial (or at least not harmful) to young children. When our newly industrialized or post–World War II economies required that middle-class women stay out of the workforce, The Voice endorsed doting care lavished by stay-at-home mothers. When affluent, highly educated women desire fulfilling careers in addition to motherhood, The Voice exalts quality time over quantity time.

The truth, as Geraldine Youcha notes in her book *Minding the*

Children: Childcare in America from Colonial Times to the Present, is that children have been successfully and unsuccessfully raised in all kinds of systems. Children have grown up as apprentices, in foster homes, in communes, in orphanages, in all-day day care, in mother-centered nuclear families, and in surrogate-centered extended families. And there are experts and professionals (and children!) who can attest to the merits and failings of any of these systems.

"The choice of one type of substitute care over another has typically been determined by prevailing values and biases more than by validated theories and empirical knowledge," Youcha writes, quoting foster care expert Anthony N. Maluccio. Youcha adds, "In the great adventure of caring for this nation's children it has not been the setting that was important, it has been the quality of care and the quality of caring."

As for me, I chose to take a decade or so out of my paraprofessional adult life in order to care for my children round-the-clock. My philosophical outlook and my skills determined that it was the right thing for me to do; my social and economic class (and a thoroughly like-minded mate) enabled me to do it.

But regardless of a child's individual family arrangement, it seems to me that an early and regular bedtime reflects, in Youcha's terms, "a quality of care and a quality of caring" that does a world of good to children growing up today. When children's basic biological need for sleep is fudged away because of the demands our workplaces make on us or because we have chosen to overlook this need, children suffer.

For the purpose of this book, then, let's assume that for whatever reason you have children and you are at home taking care of them. Or that you work on an assembly line and you're home by three every day to meet the school bus. Or that your mother takes the kids after school until you get home at five-thirty. Or that you home school. Or that you're a teacher yourself. Or that you work at home. Or that you are willing to pick them up at day care and get right to the end of the day. This book is simply a good faith attempt to set forth a model schedule that you or your surrogate can follow.

Chapter 1 will address in greater depth the reasons for adopting an early schedule for your family. Chapter 2 will chart the flow of the day—hour by hour—leading up to bedtime. Chapter 3 will detail how to cope with the exceptional days mentioned above, days when holidays, illness, travel, vacation, and special events throw a wrench into the schedule. Chapter 4 will describe some of the ramifications of the 7 o'clock bedtime and detail strategies that can actively support your rhythm in everyday life. Chapter 5 includes kitchen management strategies and recipes I've found useful when planning and preparing meals week in and week out. The bibliography lists books that have given me practical and theoretical support as I have faced the demands of all aspects of child rearing. It's my hope that these selections will provide you with the information you need to defend yourself when, as they surely will, all your friends mock you.

1

Why Bother?
(Or, Honestly, Isn't 7 O'clock a
Little Too Early?)

Nancy Birkenmeier is a nurse with the Unity Sleep Medicine and Research Center at St. Luke's Hospital in St. Louis. Over the course of 1999 and 2000, says Birkenmeier, the center received an increasing number of calls from preschool and elementary school teachers concerned about children falling asleep during school hours.

"It's very, very scary," Birkenmeier says of the trend. "The kids start having trouble going to sleep, and bedtime gets pushed later and later. Ultimately, older children start sleeping late and arriving late to school. They have trouble getting their work done, and some, eventually, drop out of school altogether. After tenth or eleventh grade the prognosis for these kids is very poor. Their parents have given up years before that, and all we can say is, 'We wish we'd gotten this kid two years ago.' "

Brown University's Judith Owens seconds the alarm: "Children between five and twelve should be the most alert people on earth," says this pediatrician, who is an associate professor of pediatrics at Brown University School of Medicine and directs the Pediatric Sleep Disorders Clinic at Hasbro Children's Hospital in Providence, Rhode Island. "When you've got children falling asleep on the school bus or in the classroom, that is a huge red flag," she says. "If you've gotten to that point, you're in serious trouble."

One experienced administrator at an independent elementary school in suburban St. Louis speaks of similar eye-opening experiences with some of the children under her watch. This professional sees children arrive at school each day suffering from the following symptoms: an inability to focus on tasks at hand; immune system weakness; reduced ability to reason; impaired memory retrieval; dysfluency (difficulty producing speech); and physical impulsiveness. She says these are all by-products of the children not getting the sleep they need, not because of any physiological malfunction like apnea (physical causes are always ruled out first), but simply because well-intentioned parents are privileging daytime activities at the expense of their children's sleep.

My husband, who for twenty years has taught English in independent high schools both in the Northeast and Midwest, adds two other symptoms of sleep deprivation he encounters regularly in his classroom. "I see a lack of creativity and a higher level of general anxiety," he says. "Of course these two things go hand in hand. When you're anxious, you cannot think creatively. These kids are just doing too much during the day."

In early 2000, Owens published a study revealing that 37 percent of the 494 suburban, middle-class children she examined suffered from at least one sleep-related problem. Teachers and parents completed Owens's survey, and the older children completed a survey on their own behalf as well. The children ranged in age from kindergarten through fourth grade. Owens says she feels her mission as a scientist and a pediatrician is to get the information before the public, both directly through the media and through her professional association with fellow pediatricians, who might do much more, she feels, to screen for sleep problems at regular checkups.

Sleep researchers like Owens and Stanford University's William C. Dement point to sleep deprivation as a significant cause of children's behavioral and learning problems. The results of current studies leave no doubt as to the consequences of compromising sleep, and the quantifiable consequences are predictably sobering.

First, a child's mood and temperament deteriorate. A chronically tired child is irritable and more easily frustrated than a well-rested child. The tired, emotionally labile child tends to overreact to his environment. Some children develop a depressive nature, losing the will or interest to participate in work and play.

Neuropsychological deficits appear next. Short-term memory falters, followed by a reduced ability to organize material. The overtired child is less able to react to situations appropriately and promptly, and loses the ability to reflect on his own behavior. He has trouble organizing his time, which leads to problems with completing homework and other personal responsibilities. These combined tasks—what scientists call "executive functioning"—reflect our highest order of cognitive thought, and are fundamentally compromised when the average child's need for sleep is compromised. I know I see enough children—my children's peers—manifesting each of these symptoms in the course of a single, average, uneventful day to make me wonder what's going on with their bedtimes.

Sadly, average children unchallenged by preexisting medical conditions are not the only children who aren't getting enough sleep. The sleep scientists I have spoken with all agree that children with intrinsic, preexisting problems like attention deficit hyperactivity disorder (ADHD) and aggressive behavior are worse off when they don't get enough sleep. Although scientists cannot yet assert that sleep deprivation actually causes these conditions, children with ADHD and hyperactivity "clearly have many more sleep problems," according to Rolanda Maxim, a developmental pediatrician and assistant professor of pediatrics at St. Louis University. Maxim explains that doctors used to believe that the medications used for treating these disorders were causing the sleep problems. Now, however, they're not so sure.

"It's very hard to say which causes which," Maxim says. "Hyper kids have a lot of noradrenaline, the neurotransmitter implicated in sleep regulation. This could be causing a whole disregulation of the central nervous system."

In early 2000 the media were abuzz with the subject of medicated children, loudly questioning how it came to be that the number of very young children taking psychotropic drugs had increased so dramatically. During this time I heard sensible voices urging people to have their children properly diagnosed before medicating them. I heard sensible voices urging parents not to assume automatically that these drugs were bad. I heard sensible voices arguing for managed care to support alternative therapies like counseling and behavior modification and not be in such a hurry for the quick fix. But I have to say that I never heard anyone, not one expert, suggest that sleep might play an important role in the cognitive and behavioral functioning of these children and their suffering families.

Amy Wolfson, associate professor of psychology at College of the Holy Cross in Worcester, Massachusetts, suggests that parents need not wait for the cause-and-effect studies to emerge before taking action. "If things are highly correlated, you take them seriously," she says.

• • •

But how much sleep is enough sleep? How much sleep does a child require in order to avoid being at risk for daytime behavior problems? Dr. John Lavigne, chief psychologist at Children's Memorial Hospital in Chicago, and Dr. Marc Weissbluth, a pediatrician and sleep researcher also in Chicago, published a study in late 1999 that examined the connection between sleep and behavior problems in children between ages two and five. Most at risk were children at age two and three who slept fewer than eleven hours in every twenty-four-hour period, these researchers found. For children four and five years old, says Dr. Lavigne, the marker was harder to pinpoint. The study did not evaluate bedtime per se, but only the total number of hours asleep in each day. Also, this study did not establish the direction of the association. The daytime problems may have been caused by the child getting too little sleep; or the daytime problems and their consequences may have done something to affect the child's sleep.

In general, though, it is helpful to have a sense of how much sleep children can be expected to require. According to the professionals at the Sleep Medicine and Research Center in St. Louis, the rough current estimates of the sleep needs of children for each twenty-four hours are as follows:

- One-year-old: fourteen hours, including one or two naps

- Two-year-old: eleven to twelve hours at night plus a single, after-lunch nap of one to two hours

- Three-year-old: twelve to twelve and a half hours

- Four-year-old: eleven and a half to twelve hours

- Five-year-old: eleven hours

- Six-year-old: ten and three-quarters to eleven hours

- Seven-year-old: ten and a half to eleven hours

- Eight-year-old: ten and a quarter to ten and three-quarters hours

- Nine-year-old: ten to ten and a third hours

- Ten through puberty: nine and three-quarters to ten hours

- Adolescent to adult: nine and a quarter hours

These numbers are guidelines only, and perfectly healthy children can sleep far less and far more than these hours suggest and still be fine. (The broad range of what constitutes "normal" sleep duration is lifelong: Adult sleep requirements can range between four and ten hours, according to Mark Mahowald, director of the Minnesota Regional Sleep Disorder Center and professor of neurology at the University of Minnesota Medical School.) The awkward years between three and five, when preschoolers are growing out of their nap but still require a certain non-negotiable amount of sleep, are a challenge to manage even for sleep mavens. Further, a child with certain chronic neurological conditions—such as forms of autism—may simply be unable to sleep for the long stretches you'd think a child would require. Consult with doctors if you are concerned. If your child does, in fact, require less sleep, there are still ways you can teach him to soothe himself alone in his room after bedtime until he is ready for sleep.

Still, given the risks of childhood sleep deprivation, it doesn't seem worth it to me to assume that your child needs a minimal amount of sleep simply because he is only getting a minimal amount of sleep. More typically, parents seem to think that their child could use a little more sleep, and never seem to worry that their child is getting too much sleep, an extremely rare phenomenon in any case.

It was the words of Marc Weissbluth that changed my life back in 1993. In *Healthy Sleep Habits, Happy Child,* he writes:

> Sleep deficiency in childhood may harm neurological development, and the problems might not show up until later. I think it is possible that unhealthy sleep habits contribute to school-related problems such as attention deficit hyperactivity disorder (ADHD) and learning disabilities. I also suspect that chronically tired children become chronically tired adults who suffer in ways we can't measure: less resiliency, less ability to cope with life's stress, less curiosity, less empathy, less playfulness. The message here is simple: Sleep is a powerful modifier of behavior, performance, and personality.

Although all humans require adequate sleep, an individual's sleep needs are a function of that individual's unique biology, psychology, and level of social interaction. From here on out, you alone will be the best diagnostician of your child's needs. The two questions you'll want to answer for yourself are: (1) How much sleep does she need? (2) When is her best moment for falling asleep? Naturally, the experts have plenty to say on both of these matters.

"Kids don't like to lie in bed awake," says Minnesota sleep specialist Mark Mahowald. This neurologist also says that there are two components of sleep that are genetically determined. One is the duration of sleep required by the individual; the other is the timing of the sleep cycle, or when those hours tend to fall in a person's twenty-four-hour day. These, of course, are the very two facts you need to establish. Mahowald, like some others I interviewed, expressed doubt that a parent might be able to modify his child's biological clock. "We fall asleep when our biological clocks permit us to go to sleep," he says. "Like eye color and height, it is a genetically determined phenomenon."

Mahowald illustrated his point by mentioning the examples of what he called sanctimonious parents complaining to pediatricians of children who are put to bed at seven o'clock but still do not fall asleep until ten. Battles erupt. Tensions run high. Bedtime becomes a nightmare. All this for no good reason, said Mahowald, who assured me that there is no clinical evidence that you can adjust your child's circadian rhythm.

If sleep onset is genetically determined, I asked, then how can a child going to bed every night at eleven possibly get enough sleep during the months and years he attends school? He cannot, Mahowald answered. And that is why he and others in the field have advocated for later high school start times, even as late as ten in the morning. In Minnesota, where public school officials have experimented with a modestly later senior high school start time (shifting first period from seven-thirty to eight), the early data suggest only favorable results.

While these studies are encouraging, not all researchers believe that the circadian clock and other intrinsic factors are entirely immune to adjustment. Mary A. Carskadon, a professor of psychiatry and human behavior at the Brown University School of Medicine and director of sleep and chronobiology research at E. P. Bradley Hospital in Rhode Island, is a leading voice in sleep research today. While Carskadon advocates for later school start times to help accommodate the special needs of adolescents, she has written that "the circadian timing system can be reset if light exposure is carefully controlled. . . . Thus we know that the system is not immutable; with time, effort, and money, we can get adolescents to realign their rhythms!" (Money, she explains, is necessary because her teenage subjects had to be paid to keep the new schedule.)

Obviously, adolescent sleep is a complicated subject. And while I do not doubt the benefits of later school starting times, I am reluctant to throw up my hands in the face of biology and rest my hopes on schools opening their doors at nine instead of seven-twenty. Mary Carskadon's work interests me because she allows for nurture's influence over nature. Dim the lights in the evening. Draw the shades at bedtime. Raise the curtains in the morning. Modify end-of-the-day activity. The biochemical apparatus of the individual sleep system, it would seem, is not entirely out of our control. Just ask any time-zone-hopping businessperson who fiddles routinely with sleep and biorhythms.

Hence the question most relevant to our purpose here is: Are morning larks and night owls born or bred? Siding entirely with either position is mostly a self-serving activity, one whose purpose is usually to justify either an action or a belief.

I tend to play it safe, and the safest (if not the easiest) place in the nature-versus-nurture debate is the gray zone. Here in the gray zone the answer to all of the above questions is "both." Larks and owls are both born and bred. But for the purposes of the 7 o'clock bedtime (as is true for any self-help guide), I am going to assume that biology is not necessarily destiny. We may be handed the tray fully loaded with all that we need for the meal, but where we sit in the cafeteria and how we eat is up to us.

Therefore, I will not consider behavior modification a doomed, hopeless, or sanctimonious endeavor. After all, I know plenty of children who don't mind lying in bed awake, and some who even like it.

Once it was believed that all children were naturally larks, up with the sun and passing the day merrily from dawn to dusk. Science and culture agreed that as children aged they grew more owlish, staying up later and later. Now, says psychologist Amy Wolfson, sleep research reveals a more nuanced picture of childhood sleepers.

According to Wolfson, not all kids are larks, although more children are larks than are owls. The owl population can be divided in two. First there are the artificial owls, those whose parents have lax or nonexistent rules regarding bedtime and what sleep expert William Dement calls sleep hygiene: the constellation of activities, behavior, and environment surrounding bedtime. These children are owls only because of what their parents are doing and not doing. Second, and this is a much smaller percentage of the gross owl number, there are the natural-born owls, children who just cannot sleep at the time that custom and culture expect that they should. Nobody knows what this number is, because many parents whose children truly belong in the first group claim that their children are in the second. The true owl child is a much rarer bird than people generally think. And finally, as we enter puberty and beyond, we all tend to move in what Wolfson called "an owl-like direction."

So here's what this means. Whether or not your children are going to bed early, most of you have larks, albeit tired larks if they're woken up for school, day in and day out. Some of you have true owls. Only a sleep specialist can tell you for sure. That's not my job. My job is to help you find a way to restore your lark's energy and joie de vivre before the inevitable shift to a later schedule occurs. If your prepubescent child is getting enough sleep, you should not have to routinely wake him up in the morning. Bedtime has to inch backward in the evening until your child wakes up on his own at the time he needs to.

If you find the responsibility of figuring out your child's clock too daunting, get help before proceeding with the 7 o'clock bedtime. There are sleep disorder centers all over the country, with staff on hand to help you. (See William C. Dement's book in the bibliography for resources.)

●   ●   ●

It may be tempting to fault sleep deprivation for a child's daytime troubles; it's less obvious, and perhaps less comfortable, to reverse the scenario: to blame our daytime choices—only one of which is the precise moment we call bedtime—for compromising her sleep. The way we live our lives has everything to do with the way we sleep. And for a child, sleep deprivation is both a cause and a symptom of life deprivation.

A child bustled along from place to place without regard for a predictable routine and reasonable bedtime is not living her own life (even if she's begging for the entertainment and activity); she is being dragged through life as if she were tied to the back of a freight train. Most likely the freight is not even her own; it belongs to the adults in her life who are pursuing an agenda of their own and preside over the engine like Casey Jones on speed. This constant hurry, this rushing headlong through life from activity to activity, ending with a period of numbing attention to the television set or to the so-called educational computer game, results in poor sleep. The poor sleep causes the daytime problems, and the cycle is kept in motion.

Donna Evans, a music teacher in St. Louis, tells the following story about a turning point in her career. Evans used to be a traditional piano teacher. One day, a young girl sitting beside her on the bench was struggling through a piece of music. Suddenly the girl stopped playing and burst into tears.

"I don't have any time to play," she cried.

Supposing that her student meant that she had no time to practice her piece for the week, Evans began to comfort her.

"No, no!" the girl cried. "I mean I have no time to play. Just play. Not piano. Play anything." And she wept inconsolably.

The girl weeping on the piano bench opened this teacher's eyes to the larger problem of hurried, harried, underrested, overscheduled children. Consequently, Evans switched tracks. Today she is no longer a traditional piano teacher but instead leads Kindermusik classes, a trademarked method through which young children come to appreciate the process of creating sound and music.

Now the last thing people need is another alarmist advocating for a fundamental change of life habits. Eat no fat! Eat no carbs! Don't smoke! Walk an hour a day! Get hip to the Internet! And while you're at it, put your kids to bed at seven! Still, that's no reason to avoid questioning our life habits. There are consequences to every choice we make, and seemingly unrelated decisions usually prove to be connected to an overall result.

Using these overarching connections, it's sometimes easier to work backward. Instead of beginning with a look at your own child's sleep habits, begin by looking at their behavior, their performance, their personality.

Open your own eyes and ears to the look and sound of your children. Are they respectful to you and to their siblings—at least most of the time? Are they alert but calm? Can they concentrate on tasks at hand? Do they fall asleep easily at night? Parents of well-rested children will answer yes.

On the other hand, if he is a preschooler, is your child inclined to have tantrums, accidents, and arguments? Does he appear unusually active or excitable? Does he tend to fall asleep in front of the television set or in the car, or on the couch in the late afternoon? Parents of overtired children may answer yes to these questions.

And what of the older children? What are they exposed to? Do they hide behind sarcasm and irony? Are they disturbingly moody? What do we expect of them, both as a culture and as individual parents? Given what we know about the needs of children, do they seem to be living lives that serve their own most profound interests? Is their way of life guiding them to be morally centered, responsible, compassionate, imaginative, loving, productive, playful, and generous members of society? Are the adults in your children's lives modeling such behavior—at least most of the time? Obviously these questions are bigger than bedtime, but they are not entirely unrelated to the daily cycles of activity and rest.

● ● ●

I turned ten in 1970, and I think ours was perhaps the first generation to really experience the earliest forms of modern overscheduling, at least in New York City, where I grew up. As one parent from that time says, "The idea was, you've got to throw a lot of paint at that canvas [meaning us kids] and see what sticks."

So I studied, in succession, cello, guitar, and piano. I swam competitively and attended religious school three times a week. My sister took gymnastics and acted in plays. (We seem downright idle when compared to contemporary kids' schedules.) When we were not doing these things we watched TV, tons of TV. Thus, in spite of the lessons, practices, and high-end secondary school homework, what seemed to stick most persistently on my own canvas were the plot twists of *I Love Lucy*, *Bewitched*, and *Good Times*.

Beginning in 1970, when our parents were divorced, my sister and I were raised by a loving, working single mother—the first in our social milieu—and we spent a lot of time on our own. Indeed, I had far more independence between the ages of eleven and seventeen than I do today with a husband and three children, a cat and a dog. I had enough independence then, I suppose, to last me a lifetime.

For thirty years parents and child-oriented businesses have fed and watered this trend, until now children of all ages are so tightly scheduled that their lives are the butt of jokes, as in "I think Max has a free hour next Monday around two-twenty." Many attitudes—fearful, hopeful, and disinterested—contribute to this circumstance.

Some parents believe that a full complement of activities beginning at birth will help their children "be all that they can be," that if the child expresses an interest in something, "you simply owe it to him to let him try it." One mother who recently sent me information concerning a gifted children's extracurricular program advised that I ought to consider such a program for my daughter because, "Heaven knows, you don't want her to be bored!"

I was too timid to reply that, yes, occasionally I do want my child to be bored. I want all my children to confront boredom, to come up against that blank wall of time and to have to find a way through that appeals to them as individuals. I do not want their lives so full and so fully planned that they never have to think about what they want to do next. (I'll elaborate on ways of coping with the overscheduling trend in chapter 4.)

Some parents overschedule their children because they fear that without that experiential edge, their children will not be competitive when the time comes to race for places in choice private secondary schools and colleges. This attitude exists despite the appeal voiced by admissions directors who prefer children who have led children's lives, and despite the virtually unanimous voices of those who care for children professionally—the teachers, school administrators, counselors, and therapists.

Marlyn McGrath Lewis, director of admissions for Harvard College, acknowledges that admissions departments are not in a position to tell parents what to do, that parental judgment and parental choice play a huge role in creating the climate of expectation in which a child matures. On the other hand, McGrath Lewis laments what she terms the "emotionally brittle" eighteen-year-old that often emerges from an overprogrammed childhood. "Children need time to become who they are," she says. "Evidence of stress and a history of being fast-tracked over time is not a plus in college admissions, at least at Harvard. We're not looking for a list of accomplishments."

Still, people doubt. One mother I know emphatically declares that admissions directors are all liars, that while paying lip service to their desire for well-rounded children, they still tend to accept those straight-A whiz kids and athletes who also profess an interest in arcane hobbies like orchid breeding and sitar playing. She may or may not be right, but I do know that to raise my children for the benefit of an evaluation that comes after twelve or eighteen years of life is out of the question. I'm not raising an Ivy League freshman; I'm raising a child.

Finally, some parents fill up their children's lives with classes and activities in order to avoid direct contact with their children, the kind of contact that is often grueling, frustrating, menial, laborious, and exhausting. Parents who allow themselves to become disengaged would rather let somebody else—practically anybody else—handle the daily grind of managing their children's behavior. This is too bad, because a disengaged parent also misses out on the payback: the beauty, the love, the warmth, and the opportunity to seize the fleeting perfect moments that don't arrive by the clock.

● ● ●

Day slides into night, and night into day. Committing yourself to the 7 o'clock bedtime means acknowledging that the way you spend your time in the light will invariably impose itself on the hours you spend in the dark.

Moreover, your goal in establishing a regular daily routine that ends at seven o'clock is not to affect perfect peace and harmony day in and day out, although you may very well manage this more often than you will believe. "Happiness, at best, is an illusory goal," writes the late child psychologist Dr. Haim G. Ginott. "It is not a destination; it is a manner of travelling. . . . It is a by-product of working, playing, loving, living." Your goal is to return your family's life to the human, to extract it wherever possible from the shabby, mercenary, competitive, philistine realm that only produces, at worst, disengaged homicidal psychopaths (think Columbine) and, at best, psychologically, sensually, and socially stunted automatons who know nothing other than how to consume facts and merchandise.

In many ways the 7 o'clock bedtime eases the road my family and I travel together. It forces us out of the mainstream, a channel I've never much admired. It forces us to be intentional about the rest of the day. And its regularity is a nightly promise that however bad the day was, it can come to an end; conversely, after a good day it reminds us that while pleasant things are hard to relinquish, part of life is letting go of what we love.

"I don't want today to end," my daughter will sometimes say to me in the dark as I head out of her room. At moments like this, I don't either. But time will not stop for either of us. All we have to hold on to is our manner of traveling, and I want her to get enough sleep for the trip. Indeed, nearly half the trip is itself that journey in the dark.

2

Time Is on Your Side:
Going by the Clock

Everyone raising children today knows that each day of the week has its own character. We schedule certain activities on certain days, which then color those days as surely as a preschooler colors blank pages with nonwashable markers. On its own, Monday has a certain personality—sometimes sad and harried after the long Sunday afternoon; other weeks fresh faced and ready to go—that is entirely different from Thursday, which I would call mindlessly routinized, with a touch of whimsy toward the afternoon as we sense that Friday is just around the corner.

This year, my two sons take after-school music classes on Monday afternoon. These classes are over by four-thirty, but the sheer length of time they must spend as responsible social beings means that a kind of time-release energy has to kick in for them all through the day. By contrast, on Wednesday the older children are dismissed from school early, at two-fifteen (my

four-year-old attends morning-only nursery school), so Wednesday tends to be a kind of carefree point of the week, when they'll
play all afternoon with each other or with friends and the time
between school and dinner seems endless.

Still, in spite of the unique nature of each school day, our
schedule overarches the week as a whole, and in fact enables the
true flavor of each day to be savored. You might consider the
schedule that follows the skeleton of your life, the bare bones that
you dress as you see fit. But just as you cannot stuff both feet into
a single boot and dance a tango, you cannot arrange your day in a
way that compromises the schedule. This schedule leaves room
for all of the variety and diversion young children require.

It is even possible, within reason and if it suits your required
wake-up times, to shift the entire schedule as a block up to an
hour later in the day, which would result in an eight o'clock bedtime. My sister's family lives a life parallel to my own, but half an
hour later; her kids go to bed at seven-thirty. This means that
every single element of her day is precisely a half hour later than
mine. She makes dinner at five, she eats at five-thirty, and so on
through the evening. If you stick to your schedule you are, after
all, establishing a circadian rhythm to your child's day, a predictable twenty-four-hour cycle of glandular, metabolic, and
sleep patterns. Think of it this way: In ordinary circumstances,
bedtime will always be two hours after you sit down to dinner.

Regularity throughout the seven days of the week is something
sleep researcher Amy Wolfson promotes, both professionally and
in her own family. Many families suspend bedtime rules on
weekends, she says, which can cause the kinds of sleep irregu-
larities that lead to trouble. This tends to happen when children
turn nine or ten years old, and are more aware of nighttime
activities. A child who stays up very late on Friday night, for example, will often pass out late on Saturday afternoon and stay up late
again on Saturday night. The same thing may happen on Sunday
afternoon, and Sunday night's bedtime may be pushed later too.

It is doubtful this child will be back on schedule by Monday morning for school.

In another scenario, children underrested from the week or from late weekend nights indulge in what Wolfson called "binge sleeping," marathon weekend catch-ups that progress far into the morning. According to Wolfson, current data suggest that a child should veer no more than sixty to ninety minutes off their weekday schedule on the weekends. That is to say that a seven-thirty bedtime should not advance beyond nine on Saturday night. You can think of these numbers working another way too. The total number of hours a child sleeps over the weekend should not swell or shrink more than sixty to ninety minutes. Parents have to keep track. Limits and rules that are sustained seven days a week (allowing for special events from time to time) guarantee that the child's biology, his circadian rhythm, functions optimally.

Beyond biology, the reward of the schedule for my children is the freedom from having to worry about what comes next. Such freedom allows them to spend their mental and emotional energy on activities and thoughts that naturally engage them. Because young children are strangers to clocks and calendars, time to them is a vast, unexplored territory that can be overwhelming. Imposing order on time soothes them and helps them relax so that they can enjoy activities in their proper time and place. Let "to everything its season" be your motto. Just after tooth brushing I've heard my four-year-old say to his older brother, "It's not the time for yo-yoing. It's book time." To a child, nothing is so incidental that it cannot warrant its own particular time of day. Their knowing the schedule also helps minimize bedtime battles, or indeed any battles over transitions. Why fight what's inexorable? Down the line, as your children come to terms with doing homework, completing household chores, or writing their own thank-you notes, their ability to structure time will serve them well.

No matter how regular you make life, however, accident and serendipity will always unsquare the corners. You always want to leave room for the occasional surprise excursion to the ice cream parlor or the unannounced trip to the zoo. But when so much is consistent in your daily routine, the spur-of-the-moment variations and surprises are appreciated for their own sake, and the accursed mess-ups are kept in perspective.

Now we will move hour by hour through the points of the day relevant to the 7 o'clock bedtime. For the schedule to progress smoothly you must keep track of the time. I don't really like wearing a watch. But ever since having kids, I wear one. I try to keep my watch checking as unnoticeable as possible; the last image you want to project is that of the White Rabbit obsessed with the time. The way to avoid this is to really see the time when you check a timepiece, and not simply glance at it absently. Try to allow enough time for transitions between activities so that you don't have to tell your children to hurry. If you give them two, five, or ten minutes of advance notice when a change is pending, then they'll be less brittle and resistant when you say "It's time to go."

"When a child is hurried," writes Dr. Ginott, "he takes his time. Most often he resents the adult's 'Hurry up!' by engaging in a slowdown. What appears as inefficiency is in reality a child's very efficient weapon against the tyranny of a timetable that is not his. Rarely should a child be told to rush."

On the other hand, after a certain age your child must be accountable for his transitions. This moment varies from child to child, but I suggest giving him some emotional responsibility beginning around age three. You will show respect for his play; he must show respect for the family's overall rhythm. This means that if you have given sufficient notice, when the moment comes for a transition, you expect the child to make it promptly and agreeably. Now must mean now. A firm statement of your expectations may be in order if he does not oblige: "I can see you don't want to go, but we have to leave now because your sister is waiting for us and we don't want to make her worry. Let's go." With these words you pick up the child (if he's not coming on his own)

and go. Ignore tears and yells. No further discussion. Remain dis-
passionate but friendly. Eventually he'll get the message: You
mean what you say. Transitions will smooth out into habit, and
the positive feedback he will garner from the other adults in his
life—carpool drivers, teachers, other parents—will help rein-
force and perpetuate the habit.

● ● ●

Although the schedule seems quite uncompromising when
described, try to imagine how it will play out in real life. Seldom
can a natural act be described in words without the description
sounding bizarre and unnatural.

If, for example, someone tried to explain to you how to eat a
thickly piled turkey club sandwich, it might sound like this: First
you take the fingers of both hands and wrap them around the top
and bottom pieces of toast, the prehensile thumbs alone supporting the two supporting pieces of toast at the base of the sandwich.
Then, as the hands bring the sandwich closer to the mouth, you
stretch your mouth open wide, wider, then even wider as your
lips take the measure of the sandwich. Next your tongue with-
draws and contracts to make room for the sandwich entry, and
finally you close the mandible so that the incisors are permitted
to slice through the successive layers of toast, mayonnaise,
turkey, bacon, lettuce, tomato, and toast.

Of course, this sounds absurdly mechanical. But that's what
language does: It gives structure to ideas, even to so sensual an
idea as the consumption of a turkey club. Thus by putting my
idea of bedtime into language you can follow I risk sounding
stilted. Understand that in reality your day will not feel like a
stylized march, even though it may read like one.

As your family's daily timekeeper, you are in a position to produce something emotionally and spiritually satisfying. Like a
conductor marking time for a multipiece ensemble, you both set

the pace and establish the overall feel of the day—fast or slow, loud or soft, urgent or expressive. You may have to reckon with more than one mood, more than one voice. One of your children may be bright and happy while the other may be low and fussy. Some of the sounds may lack harmony or be downright cacophonous. Nevertheless, it's your job to make the voices come together, or to find a way for them to separate in peace. With this simple tool of a schedule, you will be scoring a work that flows in many voices through time. I like to think of the day as music, and family life as a symphony. Here's the program:

Schedule Overview

- 6:30 to 7:30 A.M.: Day begins. Breakfast is served.

- 8:00 A.M. to 3:00 P.M.: An average school day.

- 3:15 to 4:30 P.M.: After-school snack, followed by playtime or weekly activity.

- 4:30 to 5:00 P.M.: Dinner preparation, homework.

- 5:00 to 6:00 P.M.: Dinnertime.

- 6:00 to 6:15 P.M.: Washing up for bed.

- 6:15 to 6:45 P.M.: Reading time, books, or oral stories.

- 6:45 to 7:00 P.M.: Bedtime ritual.

- 7:00 P.M.: Lights out.

6:30 to 7:30 A.M.

I don't like to wake up my children, to watch their faces go from placid and flushed to cranky and disoriented, or even benignly surprised. Mostly this is because, in a profound sense, I respect their sleep. I think it is important for them to dream, to lie undisturbed for long stretches of time, and to remain unconscious as long as their bodies require. A direct benefit of the early bedtime is that your children will awaken on their own, at the precise moment that is right for them. They will be able to lie in bed blinking and thinking for several moments, even a few minutes, before completing their daily transition from dreaminess to wakefulness.

Of course some kids awaken and leap out of bed like soldiers at the front suddenly under fire. Others need more time. But if your child is falling asleep around seven o'clock either mode is possible, because most children will not sleep longer than a dozen hours and, depending on what time school starts, will have plenty of time to get their act together before breakfast.

My ten-year-old, for example, rises around five-thirty. The house is absolutely still at this time. She reads. She does her homework. She communes with our cat. Typically she does not require my help with homework, but if she did, I would drag myself out of bed and help her. She knows she has until seven o'clock to do whatever she likes in her room. And because she is the kind of person she is, she likes peace and quiet. Which means I leave her alone. But if she were a different kind of child, I might get up every morning and chat with her in her bed or play a quiet game. After all, I have until six-thirty. At seven, everybody is due in the kitchen for breakfast.

At six-thirty my daughter comes into my room and wakes me up. This is her responsibility, a chore like any other. To her it's a chore; to me it's a luxury, since I do not like being awakened by an alarm or music. My child's morning kiss, or even her brusque pat on my shoulder, brings the night full circle. I tuck her in bed at night; she rousts me out of bed in the morning.

After swiftly dressing I go to my sons' room and kiss them if they're awake. (If anyone is still asleep I go downstairs as quietly as I can.) Then I proceed to the kitchen to empty the dishwasher and prepare breakfast. Because I tend to rely on old standbys, almost every winter morning I make oatmeal, which I serve with some kind of fruit on the side—sliced apple or grapefruit. If I'm not driving the carpool I may get a little fancy and produce fried eggs and toast, or cream of wheat, or French toast. But believe me, I am no Martha Stewart (who, by the way, is said to live on four hours of sleep a day). My goal is to fill their stomachs with something solid and sustaining that at least tips a hat to each of the food groups. I buy cold cereals of all different grains, and breads equally wholesome. At seven we all sit down and eat breakfast together.

Breakfast time is often fairly quiet. Usually the two older children come to the counter with a book (breakfast is the only meal at which I permit reading), and my four-year-old and I talk. But if the youngest seems content to chew and think, we eat in silence. Maybe I'll look at the newspaper. We do not keep our television in the kitchen (it's parked in an out-of-the-way corner of the house) and never have. So it would never occur to our kids to watch television during breakfast, as so many of their peers do. (I'll describe how we handle television in chapter 4.)

At this point you may wonder, "Where's that father, the English teacher who teaches the tired teenagers?" Most mornings my husband is out of bed by five and out the door for school sometime before six-thirty, when I arrive in the kitchen. On some mornings he plays ice hockey before school and is gone even earlier. From time to time I awaken under a lucky star because he is still in bed. Then, romantically as I can, I inquire whether or not he can drive the morning carpool. Sometimes, languid with sleep, he says yes, if in exchange I will prepare his coffee and include him in breakfast. A deal is struck. I am thrilled because now the four-year-old has no need to get up and go, and he and I can move more leisurely through the next hour or so. These are the kinds of marital negotiations that I would call win-win.

At seven-fifteen I clear the dishes (with their help) and load the dishwasher: Now the children will use the bathroom if necessary and brush their teeth. (I know a woman who, to make the morning routine even easier, keeps an extra set of toothbrushes and a tube of toothpaste by the kitchen sink.) At seven-twenty they proceed to their cubbies (each child has a couple of hooks, a shelf, and a crate near the kitchen for their backpacks and outerwear) to don shoes and coats. At seven-thirty we're out the door and driving to school. We have fifteen minutes in the car for talking before they're at the curb of school, where my two older children are due between seven forty-five and eight. (If it's my carpooling day off, I send them off at seven-thirty with a kiss and a wave, happy on the threshold in my nightgown and sweatshirt.)

Whether you chauffeur your children to and from school, or they take the school bus, your children probably spend a significant amount of time each day simply in transit from one place to another. As you imagine the course of the day, try to think seriously about the quality of life experienced by your children in these moments. If they're with you, try to be aware of what's going on behind you as you drive. Do they like to talk? Do they like to gaze out the window in silence? Do they like to read? Do they prefer listening to music? Do they like to talk with each other and you? Do they like to be quizzed on their math facts or read road signs aloud? Each day is probably different, and you can tell the minute you're all in the car how the ride's going to be. If they ride in a carpool with another family, do they generally enjoy the experience? If they ride the school bus, how do they feel about the commute? If you walk your children to school, do you hold hands and talk or do you spend the time on your cell phone? However your children get around, talk to them about what life is like for them in transit. Many adults and children enjoy the enforced downtime of the daily commute, but some can find it oppressive. Figure out what's going on in your own circumstances, and try to help your children form strategies for coping with what may be a challenging time of their day.

In our lives, preschool begins a full hour later then elementary school. If I've driven the early shift, my younger son and I may spend the hour at the grocery store, at a park, or even at a café where we'll treat ourselves to hot chocolate. After this break I move toward my second school start time, swinging by my neighbors' houses to pick up two more preschoolers. (If it's my day off, my son and I will simply return home right after the early shift. He plays until the other driver comes to pick him up.)

But these are the technical details of the morning schedule. The point is, I only see my older children for one single hour in the morning. That's all. So I'd rather make this hour as unharried as possible. Of course there are mornings that feel a little rushed. I may oversleep if my daughter forgets to wake me. A child may need a bit more than twelve hours of sleep and put the squeeze on breakfast time. (I almost never wake up a sleeping child. Just one look at that face, eyes twitching behind closed lids in the REM stage signaling that a natural awakening is imminent, turns me on my heel.) My four-year-old may rise in a funk and require extra help with dressing.

Every so often we all arrive in the kitchen and my husband is there eating his breakfast and going over the material for that day's classes. A teacher's day always begins under pressure, and my husband uses this morning hour to focus his mind and ready his spirit. For this reason, and with his blessing, I have found it easiest to act as though he is not there. We all greet him with affection, but he is in his own world and the rest of us are in ours. I do not do anything for my husband at this moment, and under normal circumstances he does not do anything for us. I have to be exuding some pretty serious SOS signals for him to hop up and tie a shoe or pour a glass of juice. After a decade of raising our family together, I have learned that I get the most annoyed when I have to ask for help that is then inadequately (to my mind) performed. It may be inadequately performed because I've not made my immediate goal clear, or because what I am asking is impossible; but for whatever reason, it is easiest on us as a couple if at certain moments I handle certain things entirely myself. (The same holds true for some of the things he asks of me, although I ignobly excuse myself on the grounds of just not liking the job he's asking me to do—say, to take a fifty-pound sack of garbage out to the alley and heave it into the Dumpster.)

Job differentiation where the children are concerned makes transitional moments much easier on them: at any given moment, one person does the zipping, lacing, collecting, searching. Even if we're going out as a family at some other time of day, generally only one of the adults is responsible for getting the children ready. "See Daddy," I will say if we're off to the park and someone approaches me with an inside-out sweater. "Right now he's in charge of getting all kids ready."

All of this raises an interesting question concerning the dual nature of a marriage that involves children. You marry someone because you enjoy their company, respect their opinions, share a sense of humor, and like experiencing life together. There is also that murky realm of your feelings and passions for each other, the realm in which intuition and anticipation see you through trouble, or get you into trouble. Your private love life lies in this realm.

Once you have children and have to face the often daunting task of unifying your collective opinions regarding raising them, it helps to cultivate a border between this murky region and the more public aspects of your relationship. This is hard, for there is a tendency to bring the murky, intuitive habits of mind to bear on child care. "She will be happy if I go get the baby and bring her into our bed because then she won't have to get up again," he may think. "Oh no," she thinks. "He only wants me to nurse in bed because he's trying to avoid sex." Never mind that he was thinking that if she were less tired she'd be more interested in sex. Murkiness reigns here, and more often than not leads a couple down the road into conflict and anguish. Meanwhile, the baby is tossing and turning in a family bed, which is kind of nice but may be getting the whole family into some pretty bad habits.

It seems to me that couples of any stripe who are raising children must eventually, if they intend to remain together over the long haul and raise decent kids, learn to separate their two ways of relating to each other. Of course there is a time and place for the shadowy muck to prevail; indeed, whether you face it openly or not it is there all the time. But there is also a time for rational, good-humored obedience to a declared policy. The health and happiness of the children, of the couple, and of the family as a whole require that both cognitive dimensions are evaluated in their proper time and place. It seems to me that the appropriate time and place for facing the muck is behind closed doors when your children are not around.

Of course fights do sometimes erupt in front of the children. I recall one embarrassing moment when, during a fight unfolding in front of the children, I actually pounded the floor with a broom to accentuate my point. Psychologists sometimes suggest that "it's even good for children to see Mommy and Daddy fight sometimes, as long as they also see the conflict resolved fairly." Personally, I've never found these performance fights very satisfying. You're always holding back, pulling punches, self-censoring for the sake of the children, and often breaking away from the argument to do a little color commentary for the nervous audience in order to clarify euphemistically what it is you're even fighting about. Allowing your children to be privy to your darkest fights on a regular basis seems a little irresponsible to me. Squabbles are squabbles, but if it's serious, it belongs behind closed doors.

Establishing policy for your family is serious, so do it alone with your spouse. Who knows what kind of baggage one of you will be carrying when it comes to sleeping arrangements? It is quite possible that dark, ancient anxieties will rear up. Separation anxiety, to name but one, is sure to be a factor when you begin to deal with sleeping arrangements. Better to get all of this out before you decide where baby is going to sleep, or whether little five-year-old Frank ought to be allowed into your bed when he has nightmares.

Once the policies are established, put them to work by the light of day. If a child introduces a problem or a contradiction in your policy, say, "You know, that's something your father/mother and I need to discuss in private. We'll get back to you as soon as we can."

When each adult (and eventually child) of the family has a reasonable set of expectations to live up to, things always go more smoothly. All of this can be managed playfully, if that is how you tend to function. Make lists of each person's duties. Put things in writing. If your children are older, draw up silly contracts with fancy names and have everybody sign them.

Perhaps this is obvious, but formal expectations do not preclude the bestowing of unplanned kindnesses and favors. I would elaborate on how my husband and I and our children tend to favor each other, but now that I think about it, it's a matter of instinct, and instincts are private. I'm sure that you can figure out how to be kind on your own, but, as I know only too well, only if you're getting enough sleep yourself!

3:15 to 4:30 P.M.

The key to an early bedtime is an early dinner. The key to an early dinner is an early after-school snack. By early I mean that your children should consume this snack as soon as school dismisses. This small repast should include something fresh and something starchy or something with a little protein. An apple and half a bagel is perfect. Fruit leather and a muffin. A yogurt and a couple of rice cakes. Cheese and crackers. A bunch of grapes and a granola bar. A handful of roasted nuts—almonds, peanuts, walnuts—mixed with raisins, sunflower seeds, and a few chocolate bits. The amount varies, depending on the kind of lunch your child eats during the day. I know my children do not consume a huge amount of their school lunch, so their snack is often pretty big by snack standards. Use your best judgment. You'll know the snack was too big if they only pick at the dinner you serve at 5 P.M. Tinker with portion size until you get it right.

If your children take the bus home, see that they have a snack in their backpacks. If you pick them up, bring it along in the car with you. If you walk them home from school, let them munch it on the way, or sit down for a few minutes near school while they eat in peace and you have a chance to talk with them. Or sit in silence.

In September 2000, the nonpartisan Urban Institute released a study of 44,000 households. The study showed that in 1997, one in five children between ages six and twelve fend for themselves during the hours between school dismissal and their parents' return from work. Children of affluent families were included in the study. Certainly, both supervised and unsupervised kids are increasingly responsible for what they eat after school. Still, even if you're not home, you can try to keep a week's worth of appropriate snacks available to them in the kitchen.

Try hard to make this snack something that they really like, because they need to understand that once they've had their snack, they are not to eat anything else until dinnertime. If they're thirsty, they can drink water. I realize this sounds a little grim, but you want them to be hungry by five o'clock or five-fifteen. Just as children cannot sleep unless they are physically and emotionally ready for bed, they cannot (or should not) be expected to eat when they are not hungry. Also, by five o'clock you will have taken the time to make a nice dinner for your family. Just as you honor a dinner party host by not eating a large bag of potato chips before leaving your house, your family honors the effort you make daily by bringing an appetite to the table.

Our circle of friends is familiar enough with our routine that our kids can be frank with other parents about our family rules.

Our four-year-old, over to play at his friend Neil's house one afternoon around four o'clock, will say to Neil's mother, "I can't have anything to eat, only water." Neil's mother, Molly, kindly obliges our system, no doubt chalking it up to my Amish-by-way-of-suburbia worldview. When she sends my children home they eat with gusto. Incidentally, we carpool with Neil's brother Sherman, who enjoys the daily snack as much as my children do. I always include him when allotting portions.

After a snack your children need to let loose and play. If they can play in a backyard or a neighborhood park, great. If the weather is bad they can play inside. You have until four-thirty to goof around. Take advantage of this time. It's a gift. Mellow or wild, the after-school playtime represents an important release from the day's demands.

Because I cherish and nurture the sibling relationships among my children, I actively protect their time alone together. I regularly say no to birthday parties on weekends and try to keep myself in the background on weekday afternoons. This is their time of day. Often they produce projects out of their backpacks to share with me, or somebody might feel the need to tell a story about the day. But generally I try to let them find their own way into the after-school hour. I look at the mail, I scan the newspaper. Left on their own, they usually get involved in something with one another—a conversation, a game, a project. After all the time they have spent in school with children their own age, they seem to fall naturally and with relief into their family configuration.

Sometimes two out of the three children will begin some activity, and the third will relish the time in solitude. One of my sons used to come home and park himself in a chair and talk to himself. If two are outside playing, the third may come in to talk to me without interruption and distraction. Some children like to pursue their private interests, whether drawing or playing with their toys.

Depending on the day, this moment in the afternoon can be extremely fragile and can therefore require serious parenting. The other day I glanced in the rearview mirror and noticed that my seven-year-old looked very worn out as we drove home from school. Suddenly he exploded in tears of sadness and rage over something that had happened over the previous weekend. He was utterly distraught, and I had to find in myself the poise to cope with him. His siblings, witnessing this outburst, realized that their brother was feeling very bad at the moment, and they quietly withdrew from the conversation. When we arrived home I suggested that he and I work together on a particular project I knew he'd enjoy. He had calmed down and was ready to move into the afternoon. A half hour of calm attention settled his soul. At bedtime that night, he said, "You know, there were two reasons I was feeling so blasted this afternoon. One was because of the problem I told you about. The other problem was that I didn't get to stretch my legs at PE today because the guys I usually play football with weren't there."

Regardless of his conclusion, I was touched by my son's effort to reflect on the cause of his breakdown, and pleased beyond words that he had the space in his life both to experience the emotion and to think about where it came from.

Some days I use this half hour to fold laundry in the same room where my children are playing. Lately, with sporadic help from my older children, I have been (unbelievably) catching up on our photo albums, currently seven years behind. I am there if they need me, and accomplishing something that I never feel like doing when I'm alone. If the chore is laundry, and the moment is right, one or more of them will help me fold and cart things off to the proper drawers.

The two things they cannot do at this time are watch television or use the computer.

If your children are engaged in any after-school activities, three-thirty to four-thirty is the ideal time to schedule them. For the moment it's enough to say that elementary school children should have no more than one such activity a week, and that this activity should be over by four-thirty at the latest if it's scheduled on a school day. If you have more than one child, the goal is to arrange all of the extracurricular activities on the same afternoon. My experience has been that this is almost impossible if you have more than two children. But it's always worth a try. This year I came awfully close, with my sons' music classes meeting concurrently on Monday afternoons and ending at four-thirty. My daughter's half-hour violin lessons are Tuesdays at three-thirty, which gives the boys and me an enforced sitting-around time in the lobby of the music school. We read, or my seven-year-old does his homework, or the two boys goof around.

Lobby time is something we all usually enjoy, but Mondays and Tuesdays are still our long days, and a feeling of tension has usually built up by the time we arrive home. For a child under ten, nine hours is a long time to be away from home. While my youngest is home alone with me between noon and three, my seven-year-old has been going full tilt. He's the one I watch for signs of fretful exhaustion. Now that he can read, I see him weathering the time between four-thirty and five o'clock more easily. He may change into sweatpants, curl up in his bed under the covers, and read until dinner. The youngest takes his cue from his brother and will climb onto his own bed to play with stuffed animals until they hear the call from me. This represents the best-case scenario; the worst case scenarios—those that involve tears, conflicts, and worries—require all the patience and insight I can marshal while simultaneously handling a cleaver.

If family life is seriously disintegrating before your eyes, it's crucial that you recognize the need to break from your activity and step in for hands-on conflict management. Good teachers intuit these moments as a matter of course. Once, on a field trip with forty fourth-graders, I witnessed such a moment. We were forty children, six or seven mothers, and four teachers hovering in front of the botanical gardens, waiting to go in. The children were barely under control—excited, talkative, bursting with energy first thing in the morning. We mothers were chatting among ourselves, awaiting the next command from one of the lead teachers. Suddenly I noticed a small commotion in the center of our crowd. One of the lead teachers drew a child out of the group's midst, led him off to the side by the shrubbery, and with a very serious expression began reprimanding him. By now the doors of the garden had been opened, but we could not make a move on our own. Clearly, a major infraction had occurred, one so pressing that in a split second the teacher determined to keep more than fifty people waiting several minutes until he had coped with the offender.

It's moments like this that make me wonder how people can say that being with babies and children turns your brain to mush. Like experienced actors doing improvisation before an audience packed with critics, people who care for children know that the stakes are always high. At any moment you might say the right or the wrong thing, make the right or the wrong move. Actors have to know what they want to accomplish in a scene; parents and teachers have to know what kinds of children they want to produce. Calculation and forethought are essential when you feel you are serving the big picture at all times. And somehow, in spite of this, what you say and what you do have to be honest and unscripted. Considering this, it's no wonder some parents would rather spend the afternoon sitting on the sidelines shouting at a ref.

Dinnertime can always be delayed if one of your children needs to learn the lesson of a lifetime.

4:30 to 5:00 P.M.

At four-thirty you need to be in the kitchen preparing dinner. If you're in the yard, come inside. (The kids can keep playing.) If you've been out and about, be home by now. This is a good time for children with homework to sit down near you and get to work. Many young children prefer tackling their worksheets with an adult nearby to help when questions arise. Others enjoy reading aloud while you prepare dinner. If anyone takes music lessons, this is the time to practice. Pour everyone a nice tall glass of water—yum! yum!—and pull the meal together.

The subject of homework for children older than seven or eight is a can of worms. To judge from recent newspaper articles and letters to the editor, it's a subject that has been increasingly inflaming educators, parents, and children. Some would like to abolish homework altogether; others view it as a mark of peda-gogical seriousness and fear that without it our children will grow dumber and less intellectually disciplined than some imag-ined foreign horde of homework-doers. Whatever your feelings on the matter, you can probably admit that completing homework is fundamentally a matter of time management. For this reason it bears directly on your afternoon and evening schedule and directly affects the 7 o'clock bedtime.

When my eldest child was in first and second grade, I worried a great deal about what I'd heard was going to be onerous loads of homework beginning in fourth grade. More than once I broached the subject with the school head, who calmly assured me that whatever homework my daughter was assigned she would be ready to take on, and that the school had built-in proto-cols for ensuring that the homework did not get out of hand. So I stopped my pestering, confident that by working with my child's teachers I could bring a halt to homework that demanded any more than an hour and a half to complete (including a half hour's reading time).

As my daughter's homework load has increased, we have kept it well within these limits. As I mentioned earlier, she generally does her hour's worth of homework alone in the early morning. (Her daily recreational reading easily surpasses the required half hour.) If a large project is coming up, she spends weekend hours working on such an assignment, anticipating that there may not be time enough during the week. Because she is a highly motivated and independent student, I do not review her work before she turns it in. If something is going wrong in either her study habits or her independent work, her teachers let us know directly through notes or conferences. If I don't hear anything, I assume all is well.

Obviously, not everyone is comfortable with this level of letting go. Trusting the process means having faith in your child and in her school. It helps to be married to a secondary school teacher, who can constantly reassure you that it's better to struggle and sometimes fail on your own than to succeed because of parental involvement. Still, there are certainly some children who may benefit from some degree of adult help. Whatever your feelings about helping with homework, you must attend to the time your child needs to complete his assignments. This is a matter of scheduling life outside of school, and will be discussed further in chapter 4 when I examine the consequences of establishing an early bedtime.

If you know that one of your children will require help with her homework on a particular night, plan ahead. Order a pizza or heat something out of the freezer. If you're home at midday, prepare a casserole or soup that you can start heating around four. Wash lettuce for a salad. Serve this with a block of cheese and a loaf of bread. Do what you have to do to avoid kitchen detail because, in order to end the day at seven o'clock, dinner has to be on the table at five. It is possible to compress the activities between dinner and bed into less than two hours, but then you will feel rushed. Two hours give you ample time to do what needs to be done in a peaceful way. So if you're not going to make dinner, somebody else has to. (Chapter 5 presents recipes for make-ahead dinners and suggests meals that can be prepared in a half hour.) And there are worse things than carry-out meals or cold cereal for supper.

I may as well remind you that children are not to watch television now, either. You may want to play some music they favor—anything they like and you can tolerate at this time of day is fine. I find that the music from certain Broadway shows—*Fiddler on the Roof, 1776, Oliver, Godspell, My Fair Lady, The Sound of Music, Pippin,* and *Oklahoma,* among others—appeals to a range of tastes in our family. The children love the catchy tunes and like to follow the stories the songs relate.

A side benefit of listening to musicals is that they frequently introduce historical episodes that usually require some unpacking on my part. Czarist Russia, colonial America, nineteenth-century London, the life of Christ, class consciousness in Edwardian England, Austria's role in World War II, the crusades of the Holy Roman Empire, and the settlement of the Wild West have all been discussed as a result of listening to the shows listed above. Teachers will say to me, "Wow, your kids seem to know a lot of history." Little do they know where this knowledge comes from. Of course, Broadway musicals are not for everyone. If musical theater sets your teeth on edge or conjures up dinner theaters in the far reaches of Long Island where you were dragged circa 1973, then there's always Raffi, whose slurry, slightly strained voice on the early albums strikes me as somewhat Dylanesque.

5:00 to 6:00 P.M.

Eating dinner at five o'clock seems totally odd, you say. Fair enough. It is a little odd. If it helps, the adults in the family can think of it as a late lunch. Indeed, working parents can leave the after-school care to another person and just show up at five as though it's a lunch break. By seven the kids are in bed and you can go back to work! To you it's a siesta. To your children it's a calm, predictable bedtime at the time that is right for them.

I realize, of course, that most parents are not schoolteachers who can put in a ten- or eleven-hour workday and still be home in time for a five o'clock dinner. Many parents do not come off assembly lines at three, do not home school, don't work the midnight shift, and do not have the flexibility in their day necessary for spending the hours between five and seven at home with their children. A child's daily needs are not necessarily easy to coordinate with the needs of the working-day world.

On the other hand, I do know working parents of both sexes who try very hard to be home in time to eat dinner with their children. Some are executives who rush away from the office each day at five and sit down to the table at five-fifteen. Others schedule their family dinners at six and find that an eight o'clock bedtime works just fine.

One thing is clear: For most parents in this day and age, a routine family dinner served at the same time every single night cannot happen without a great deal of compromise on everyone's part. Cut short that afternoon meeting; tear yourself away from the gossip at the watercooler; pack up the briefcase and plan on doing the work at seven-thirty, after bedtime. These are just some examples of the compromises I know parents make for the sake of dinnertime. You have to ask yourself whether you really cannot be home by five o'clock, or whether it's just too inconvenient to arrange your work in order to do so. (In chapter 4, I'll address the afternoon compromises made by the rest of family.)

From the perspective of the family's primary caregiver, there are other considerations to weigh. For instance, what happens when the phone rings in the kitchen at five o'clock?

"Hi! It's me. Listen, I got caught up in a meeting and can't get out before five-thirty. There's no way I'll be home before six."

"I'm sorry to hear that," says the person at home with the children. "We'll go ahead and eat and see you at six."

Family dinner is family dinner. Very young children cannot be expected to eat a few canapés and make small talk while waiting for that parent who's running late. What if there's traffic? What if the meeting goes on and on because the boss is avoiding a return to his own unhappy home? Sit down with your kids and eat, and the missing parent will catch up with the routine when he or she finally gets home.

I know many women whose husbands travel on business all week long. Almost unanimously, these women say that the evening and bedtime hours are unbelievably easier—more relaxed, more pleasant—when their husbands are not around. Dinner can be served at the time that is right for the children, which automatically brings bedtime into line. One parent at home with the children will naturally short circuit the likelihood of an evening witching hour. Often it's only a matter of shifting dinner earlier by fifteen or twenty minutes, something a stay-at-home caregiver is reluctant to do when the whole family is waiting for the grand moment when Mr. or Mrs. Breadwinner walks in the door.

A five o'clock family dinner makes conversation possible. Young children are not so strung out that they ruin the meal for everyone. Older children are usually happy to talk at this hour. Parents can maintain order at the table yet allow the children to have their say. In theory, I ought to have said, this moment comes together in this way. But in reality, familywide conversations sometimes work and sometimes don't.

The biggest behavioral issue in our family concerns interrupting. Everyone has something to say and everyone has a hard time waiting his or her turn. When I ask our four-year-old to please wait his turn to speak, he says, "I'm afraid I'll forget what I was going to say." He's got a valid point, so I'll have to wait for some inspiration before I make him a proper reply. I can't bring myself to say what we've all heard—"If it's really important it will come back to you"—because I know from experience it often doesn't come back to you, at least not right then. Should we account for the relative capacity of individual memories when allotting turns to communicate? I'm not quite sure yet. I think someone ought to write a book about interrupting.

The other night I was so frustrated by our youngest's whining and interrupting as we sat down to dinner that I told him that he needed to be absolutely quiet, absolutely totally quiet. He was not allowed to say anything at all. All he could do was chew until I said he could speak again. Oddly enough, he complied with nary a protest. He sat and ate contentedly, as though somebody had defused a bomb inside him, even going so far as to hand-signal to me when he wanted some more applesauce rather than make the request aloud. If anything, he seemed relieved to no longer be the nexus of so much irritation. It was his brother who lobbied me instead: "But, Mommy, what about that law you were talking about the other day?"

"What law?"

"The law you were talking about. About those guys in the white hoods."

Ah! he was referring to our conversation about the Ku Klux Klan and their right to clean up a section of a local highway. Freedom of speech and all that. So, as the youngest sat silently, consuming applesauce by the jarful, my husband launched into a reply about using good judgment about our speech, and knowing when to speak and when not to speak, and many other aspects of the subject. The moment was proof positive that, however unpleasant and frustrating dinnertime moments can sometimes start off, they are certainly learning experiences. One moment you're reminding someone to use a fork. The next moment you're airing your views on freedom of speech.

At dinner your children witness your own efforts to be polite. My husband thanks me for making dinner. If he's made the dinner, I thank him. Even if the meal is lousy, we try to find one kind thing to say about it. Always, I try to hold the ideal dinnertime in my imagination, and I work night after night to bring my family into line with this ideal, with more and less success. Some nights are just plain awful, and I excuse everyone with relief when the meal is over. But no matter what kind of a dinnertime we experience, I do feel that the moment is a cornerstone of our daily life.

I have a friend whose husband runs the dinner table conversa-

tion. She says that since she's been with the children all afternoon, she has no need for news. She's worn out from the day and
has no stamina left to guide conversation. Her husband, on the
other hand, is home from work and ready for data. He will ask
each of the children to name five things that happened to them in
school that day. And they oblige. According to their mother, his
energy and interest inspires them to take mental notes throughout the day so they'll have items to share with him at dinner. This
method would never work in my family. Our kids tend to clam up
if they feel they're under interrogation. Moreover, my husband
has been providing and summoning the vitality for classrooms of
adolescents all day. He's not generally capable of eliciting even
one more comment.

Sure, dinnertime is for eating and, fleetingly, for adult conversation. But dinnertime can also be viewed as an extremely important moment in the social development of the human. We all
exchange information and tell stories, my husband and I connect
with each other, the children observe this connection, and they
are taught (over and over again) how to participate in a group
conversation. When people talk about the work involved in parenting, family dinners with young children are the kind of thing
they're talking about. And sometimes, just sometimes, the ideal is
made real. A subject is introduced and the children are engaged
in it, and they are not too tired or too hungry or too antsy to sit
through the discussion and have it spark their thoughts into
flame.

The other night our ten-year-old told us about a classmate who
had sprained his ankle that afternoon and had to go home in the
middle of the day. This triggered a discussion about accidents,
crutches, and stitches—things our children tend to regard with
a kind of wide-eyed, awful attention. So my husband was urged
to recount all the times he was on crutches, which led to a couple
of long stories involving racing afoot through root-filled under-
brush. Our eldest child mentioned her recent stitches (for a deep

cut she gave herself while whittling a stick), and our seven-year-old mentioned his affair with crutches, when he had badly banged his toe into a baseboard. Landing on a subject that permits almost everyone to contribute is like stumbling upon a gold nugget in the aisle of the grocery store. When it happens, be grateful and do not cut it short, even if this means stretching out dinner past your scheduled time. Herein lies the art of successful parenting: knowing which waves to ride and which to let pass.

In order to ride the unexpected conversational wave, it is very important not to answer the telephone during dinnertime. In general, regard the telephone as inimical to family life. We have come to accept all kinds of rude interruptions to the peace of a family circle; telephone use is one area we can control. I've toyed with the idea of declaring up to one hour a day for placing, returning, and receiving calls, somewhat like a monarch presiding over an open court for a limited time each day. Children who tend to resent any time you spend on the phone would, I think, come to accept this as a compromise and leave you in peace as long as you honored the deal. With respect to meals, it would be best to shut off all ringers, so that you don't even have to spend a thought on wondering who had just called.

Plan to stay at the table until five-forty-five or so. After the main course, let the children clear the table while the adults serve dessert, which can range from fruit to pudding to a scoop of sorbet to orange slices. The flow from course to course is a challenging ritual, and the children learn a little bit more about coping with civilization.

Following dessert, or after the main course if there is no dessert, our children ask to be excused before clearing what they can from the table and going about their business. A formal conclusion to the meal helps mark the moment when the official hour of bedtime arrives.

At this point, one of the adults does the dishes while the other takes the children off to wash up for bed. If the dishes are done in ten or fifteen minutes, the dishwasher can then take one of the kids for a one-on-one book time. Or manage the baby (if there is a baby) while you put the older kids to bed. Let the baby stay in his high chair fingering Cheerios while the dishes are getting done. In order to get the dishes done, it helps to know just how long your baby can sit in a high chair without fussing. If necessary, you can always do them after bedtime, but this is something I try to avoid.

If you are a single parent or your spouse is unavailable, you may excuse yourself from the table a little prematurely in order to have the dishes clean by six.

Lately our sons scamper upstairs for ten or fifteen minutes of play (Warning: Do not try this at home yet. Our kids are so thoroughly immersed in the schedule that we can give the boys a free rein at this moment. They know that when either parent appears in their room, it's time for tooth brushing and face-and-hand washing. One pleasant but firm announcement usually brings them to the sink.) Meanwhile, my husband and I clean in the kitchen with our ten-year-old for company. For me, this time alone with my daughter and my husband seems miraculous. I can imagine that for her it feels very special too, although I don't want to break the spell by asking her about it. Often she's happy to sit and eavesdrop on our conversation, which can adjust to another level with the younger set out of the room. Other evenings she has more to offer about her day or things in general.

6:00 to 6:10 P.M.

Around six o'clock you're in the bathroom with your children, brushing their teeth and helping them wash up. Your big, calm body reassures them that this is going to happen because you are right there to make it happen. Always try to avoid the kinds of shooing-off commands such as "run along and brush your teeth now" that distance you from the hands-on care of young children. Even midmorning, when most children are at the peak of their day's energy, staying on task is a challenge. It's not really fair at their most emotionally vulnerable time of day to expect young children not to veer off into some other appealing activity on their way to the bathroom. If you send your children upstairs after saying that you'll join them "in just a second as soon as I get this kitchen cleaned up," chances are by the time you arrive in their room one child will be flipping through a book and the other will be adding a few pieces to a Lego compound and you'll have to end what has turned into a playtime.

I know of a dentist who still brushes his fourteen-year-old daughter's teeth because he's convinced kids don't do a good enough job on their own. This may or may not be true, but you can always ask your dentist if your children's teeth are getting properly cleaned. Of course, children under five or so still need you to do it for them—after they've had their own turn. Usually I enjoy brushing my four-year-old's teeth. But sometimes he is really all done in, and I must scoop him up into my arms and carry him into the bathroom. I do this as calmly as I can, trying to ignore his screams. I balance my left foot on the rim of the bath-tub and perch him on my thigh with my left arm around his waist. I prepare the toothbrush and set to brushing. Actually, an open yelling mouth is quite easy to clean. And I know my child. Some-times he just has to blow off steam. Fortunately, the only thing he can harm at this close range is my eardrum. Usually he doesn't wriggle or fight to escape, but even if he does, I am stronger than he. By the time we're done, he's usually settled down, or at least whimperingly heading for the bureau, where I get him into his pajamas.

Try to get all of your children to shower or bathe on the same night. This is important, because then on bath night you can plan to end dinnertime at five-thirty or five-forty, which will give them enough time to play in the tub or to enjoy an unrushed shower. In the wintertime, assuming they've not done anything that has made them really dirty, our kids bathe or shower once a week.

Babies and toddlers require more frequent bathing, both for the sake of hygiene and so that they can play freely in warm water.

Much as the following admission will shock and dismay my own mother, I've never really seen the need for daily baths for children over three who have not reached puberty. If it's something your family does because bath time gives your children immense pleasure, or because it winds them down for the day, or because you feel they must wash their entire bodies more often, that's fine. And there are all kinds of ways of fitting bath time into your schedule. In one family I know the children shower in the morning before breakfast. Their mother says that this wakes them up and makes them feel ready for a new day. Some afternoons I draw playtime baths for my sons at four-thirty, and they come down to dinner clean and fresh.

Depending on how long you spend at dinner, you can have as much as a half hour (five-forty-five to six-fifteen) for the washing time. I tend to take extra time for reading at the expense of bathing, but this is a matter of personal taste and the stage of your children. When they were very young, my children sometimes spent an hour in the tub. How you manage the transition from mealtime to washing time is up to you. It's another place where the schedule can be tweaked to suit your own family.

Usually, we try to bathe or shower our children late on Sunday afternoon. There is less pressure that night because the children are rested from the weekend. But if a bath is needed during the week and if for some reason we're running a little late, I'll sometimes read to my sons while they relax in the tub. In *Parenting as a Spiritual Journey*, Rabbi Nancy Fuchs-Kreimer speaks of bath time (and every other time of day) as potentially sacred time. "It is a time for soaking away the stains of the day (or sometimes the week)," she writes, "watching our children becoming clean, fresh, and pure once again. As we wash away our children's grime, we can let ourselves believe that our hearts, too, may become clean again."

During the summer our children shower daily because they have to wash off the day's worth of chlorine, sunscreen, and sweat. But when school's out there is less pressure on the evening in general. We'll have a closer look at vacations in chapter 3.

Between six and six-fifteen everyone is climbing into pajamas—with or without help—and selecting their bedtime stories.

6:15 to 6:45 P.M.

No later than six-fifteen you are lying on your big bed, or on one of their twin beds, or on the floor, or anywhere that you and they are comfortable. Read to them, make up a story, or tell them something about your life when you were little. This is not the time to tell them about the time you got locked in the bathroom on an airplane and called for help and nobody came in spite of your pounding on the doors and screaming. Nor should you relate to them your memory of the time the repo man came and took away your dad's car. Make the remembrance something simple and comforting, perhaps something about your favorite holiday and how it was celebrated, or about a birthday you really loved and remember well. Or maybe you once lost something special to you and then found it again. The simplicity of the narratives that appeal to children is amazing. The story doesn't have to be a happy one, though, if it's poignant and contributes to your child's mental picture of you as a child.

Rahima Baldwin Dancy, in *You Are Your Child's First Teacher*, writes that "when you tell a story, you weave a magic web in which the listeners become engrossed, and there is nothing between you and the children to distract your attention or theirs. By telling the story instead of reading it, you are also free to note the effect the story might be having on the child."

Fuchs-Kreimer also notes the importance of storytelling: "Narrative theologians explain in fancy language what primitive people, children, and parents already know. Before there were dogmas and rules, there were stories. Fundamental to any religion, any life, is the shaping of raw experience through story, giving narrative form and meaning to events. Stories provide a structure for understanding the world."

I remember loving a story my mother used to tell about being forgotten at ballet school one snowy afternoon. Nobody had come to pick her up, and she'd had to walk all the way home by herself. When she arrived home, there were bits of snow and ice on her eyelashes from the tears she had shed along the way. Most dramatic and disturbing was the part where she walked into the warm house and found her mother, father, and brother already at the table eating dinner. She hadn't even been missed! Very strange.

She also used to tell us about the time she went on a teen tour through the Canadian Rockies. In order to explore the crags and precipices of those picturesque mountains my mother and her fellow teens were mounted on well-stepping horses. After days of navigating switchbacks and spine-chilling descents, my mother learned that her horse was in fact blind. Of course I knew she had survived (her living flesh was sitting on my bed), but the sheer drama of the story always gripped me and made me feel my mother was somehow both vulnerable and lucky.

My father, on the other hand, tended to make up stories. I'll spare you the details of the ongoing adventures of Joe and Flo but will admit that their home life (which takes place "on the outskirts of Baltimore") and their idiosyncratic family members have been brought into the new millennium with very little modification of the story's basic structure and characters. Neighbors and pals, Joe and Flo wake up each morning and in their respective homes eat Rabelaisian quantities of breakfast foods, usually ending the meal with something like one grape. Then they go off together, to the circus, to the park, to a hill for sledding. They encounter a few wacky characters along the way, help out where they can, and return home for gargantuan suppers and, of course, bed. For obvious reasons, my stories almost always end with the characters going to sleep.

Making up a story for your children is one of the most rewarding experiences you can have. Sometimes you stumble upon a plot that somehow manages to dazzle, amuse, and instruct them, and you leave their room feeling nothing less than Dickensian. But even if the story falls completely flat to your ears, to your children it is like a small miracle. Moreover, you will know soon enough whether the story was a hit or a flop: no waiting around for the morning papers. If it was good (and by "good" I mean if the story somehow spoke to them in a highly meaningful way) they'll ask for it again the next night, or for a sequel. If they ask for a book, then you know your narrative was missing something they needed.

"For a story truly to hold the child's attention," writes Bruno Bettelheim in *The Uses of Enchantment,* "it must entertain him and arouse his curiosity. But to enrich his life, it must stimulate his imagination; help him to develop his intellect and to clarify his emotions; be attuned to his anxieties and aspirations; give full recognition to his difficulties, while at the same time suggesting solutions to the problems which perturb him."

Sounds like a tall order. On the other hand, you know your child better than anyone. You know exactly the kinds of things she is curious about. You know what she tends to worry about. You know what she hopes for. You know what she struggles with day to day. You know what makes her happy. A child under seven or so can be told a story about herself that is entirely encoded so that she does not consciously realize what you are up to. If you are interested in attempting a story of this kind, simply make the protagonist an animal or a child with a different name or gender.

Say your child is selective about what he eats. Make up a story about a little boy who only ate—you name it—frozen peas. Make it sound perfectly reasonable. Frozen peas, why not? His mother put only frozen peas in his lunch box. He ate frozen peas after school. For breakfast he ate frozen peas with brown sugar until . . . what would happen to him? Maybe he finally got bored and switched to frozen corn. The only thing you cannot do is draw an explicit likeness between your story's character and your child. For the story to be fun, it has to occupy a place where your child is entirely unaccountable. Stories do most of their magic subliminally.

It's easiest, however, to tell stories with no apparent agenda. Here's how. First, demand that the room be as dark as possible so that you can think up the words. Everyone gets as comfortable as possible and tries not to wriggle. Then you begin, as ever, with "Once upon a time there was." If you feel like creating an interactive narrative, you inflect your sentences at key moments, which invites your child's contribution as follows:

You: Once upon a time there was a little . . .

Child: Kangaroo. [Bear, frog, piece of paper, girl]

You: Who lived in Australia with her mother and father and brother. And the little kangaroo's name was . . .

Child: Blinky. [Sarah, Kitkat, Juicy, George]

You: Blinky. And one day Blinky decided to go out and see what was happening at the lake. So she asked her mother if she could go, and her mother said, "Of course, just be back by lunchtime." So off she went.

And you're off. Maybe a dingo was prowling around the lake and Blinky has to figure out a way to warn her friend Jonah that a dingo is nearby. Jonah, a neighbor kangaroo, has been doing some reckless things lately, and Blinky is trying to figure out what she can do to stop him. And so on. Really, anybody can tell a story. Feel free to have characters who misbehave and require your child's interjections to straighten out the misbehavior. You can interrupt yourself and ask your child if he thinks it was wise of Blinky to take on such a big problem without help. Or maybe Blinky goes off to the lake and meets a really friendly wombat, who takes her to his home and introduces her to all kinds of wombat ways of life. She returns home with some stories of her own to share with her mother.

By such simple means you show your children that storytelling is a natural human activity, one that you do not need a special license, degree, or Hollywood contract to practice. Anyone can do it.

Incidentally, you do not have to invite your child's participation in the story. Some children (and narrators) prefer that one person only take authorial responsibility for the narrative.

You never know where an idea will come from. One evening many years ago, as we sat at the dinner table with my parents, the children's grandfather mentioned something about the Texas Rangers. My then three-year-old was fascinated, but I was a little worried that the gunslinging legends might haunt his dreams. At some point within a few weeks I introduced a bedtime story about some Texas Rangers of my own. Somehow the story worked, and the plot—which involved cattle rustlers altering stolen steers' brands by adding bars to each hide, thereby turning *L*s into *E*s—was a major hit. Half a decade later I'm still telling Texas Ranger stories by command performance. Mind you, I know nothing whatsoever about the real Texas Rangers. And not once, in all my stories, has a pistol (or whatever the gun was that they slinged) been fired.

When in doubt, bring something to life. There's a reason Pinocchio and Frosty the Snowman are immortal. Maybe one day Sally woke up and found her stuffed bear in the kitchen eating a bowl of cornflakes. Then she has to spend the rest of the day keeping the bear out of trouble. Or say you're a mechanic: One day you get to work and discover your tools building something on their own. Now, for a change, the mechanic has to do whatever the tools say.

One last thing about making up your own story: feel free to steal mercilessly from stories you have heard before. Trust me, your kids won't sue you for plagiarism. In any case, the words coming out of your mouth are yours. If you want to tell a story called "Sam and the Three Aardvarks" instead of "Goldilocks and the Three Bears," go right ahead. Little Sam will probably love it, and you won't have to spend any energy on plot spinning.

But what if you're so tired by bedtime that the very thought of thinking up anything at all pushes you over the edge? Try a story about someone who goes to sleep. There's always Sleeping Beauty and Rip Van Winkle. Then you can lie there silently for a few minutes, mock snoring perhaps, when you get to the part where the hero/heroine's asleep. If you're asked, you can call this dramatic realism. Take as long as you can get before your child prompts you to continue.

Story time usually lasts thirty minutes or so, until about six-forty-five. Children who read on their own do so at this time too.

If you finish the book or story time with minutes to spare, turn off the lights and see what happens. Some kids will open up to conversation at this time of day only. Young children may feel the need to comment on something about the story. Older children may need to tell you something that happened at school that they couldn't really put into words earlier.

When my daughter was very young, beginning around age three, we began keeping a journal, making entries at this time of day. Often, because I was juggling her infant brother on my lap, it was nearly impossible to maintain control of the pencil and the little notebook. Most of the entries reported that she had played with her friend Maria in the afternoon, and that she had "felt happy all day" but now felt "really tired. And that's all for the day." This business about feeling happy resulted from my trying to explain that a journal didn't have to record only activities, but also feelings, that it was a way to keep track of what you had been feeling as you grew up. But she was truly so tired, and so young, that even a fit suffered earlier that day was ancient history.

Once she could write on her own, my daughter kept her journal on again and off again for a couple of years. Now she returns to the practice every so often. Our first-grader has been keeping a journal more or less since he was four. Like his sister's, it began with my husband or I taking dictation, but it has evolved now into his own, truly private realm.

Even without a journal, this moment when the lights go off lends itself quite naturally to thoughtfulness and reflection. If somebody else has managed your child's day up until six o'clock when you walk in the door, a focused, loving story time and quiet time every single day builds up an enormous amount of love and trust between you and your child.

6:45 to 7:00 P.M.

After book time everyone gets into their own bed. Here is where you custom design the closing moments of the day. What rituals mean something to you? How do you want to send your kids off to sleep every night? If you say prayers, now's the time for prayers. If you lower the shades, now's the time to lower the shades. (During the winter, when it's dark at seven o'clock, pulling the shades is more a ritual than a necessity. In early fall, spring, and summer there is still some daylight outside, and pulling the shades is more important. A darkened room helps convey the idea that it's time to sleep. Scientists talk about the light sensitivity of the pineal gland and the brain's need for darkness in order to allow sleep a purchase. Common sense says pulling the shades helps turn a bedroom into a sleeping room. Even babies can yank on a shade pull every night. It's a hands-on way of saying good night to the world.)

If you switch on night-lights, now's the time. If you like to sing lullabies, now's the time to sing. The important thing is that all of these last steps are done in the same order, in the same way, every single night. And you really can establish the pattern as early in the life of the child as you wish. Begin as soon as you come home from the hospital and are able to walk around without the postpartum limp. Because while you may or may not be training your newborn to expect predictable patterns, you most definitely are training yourself. You have a child now, and you may as well get yourself used to what the routine will be like for the next dozen or so years. (Newborns don't go to bed at seven o'clock. For them, the most important thing is making the pattern routine, not sticking to the clock.)

When our first child was a baby I was completely flummoxed for several months. I nursed her constantly, never let her cry for any reason without trying to comfort her, and tried to establish her bedtime at seven o'clock from the time she was tiny. Which meant that when she finally did consolidate her sleep, that first chunk was seven to midnight instead of eleven at night to four in the morning. For this reason my own sleep was thoroughly wrecked. I was exhausted, irritable, and borderline demented. Throughout our daughter's infancy, my husband and I stumbled along using one system after another until we fell back on the routine that had seen us through the roughest times, namely, my husband walking the baby back and forth behind our house—sometimes for an hour or more—until she finally stopped watching the trees go by and conked out on his shoulder.

On the eve of the Persian Gulf war, when she was fourteen months old, my husband and I tried training her to sleep using the notorious Ferber method. Following the directions spelled out in Dr. Ferber's book, I put our daughter down in her crib while she was still wide awake but ready for bed. She cried. After a minute I returned, gave her a pat, said "night-night," and left the room again. She cried. In our room my husband and I huddled over the transistor radio listening to the developments in Kuwait. Two minutes later I returned to my daughter's room, gave her another soothing pat, then left again. She continued to cry. We increased the minutes between the pats until finally, after at least an hour of crying without interruption, she fell asleep. It was a trying night for all of us. Ultimately, neither the war nor the method worked out exactly as planned, but this mission did mark the dawn of my respect for her schedule as her nights and naps fell into predictable order.

Our bedtime ritual really began before then, though, when she was perhaps six months old and eating solid food. Dinner at six, bath at six-forty-five, book time at seven-fifteen. Following book time we'd go over to the window, say good night to all the things we saw out the window, pull down the shade, turn off the light, and walk up and down her tiny nursery. I held her in my arms and told her quietly about what she'd done that day. Then I'd sing one song and settle down in the big chair to nurse her. If she fell asleep nursing, fine. If she didn't, I'd put her in her crib and she had to fall asleep on her own.

Things often got a little hairy here if she wouldn't go to sleep in her crib. And although we made a bunch of mistakes with our first child, the sense of a bedtime routine certainly began at this time. With each of our successive children we improved our technique, and by the time our third child came along the final moments of bedtime had become pleasant instead of horrible.

I know one father who pulls out his guitar and sings to his children as they lie in bed. Another mother scratches backs. Massaging your child before sleep—especially his hands and face—is something you can do while you sing. Apart from establishing your presence, it physically relaxes the child. Some people kiss their child's palm, then tell the child to place the palm on their cheek if they feel lonesome in bed. You might tuck in stuffed animals, or blow out the candle that you'd lit for the story time. After the rituals, you declare your love, kiss and hug them, and say good night.

Some people are comfortable just walking out the door and letting the kids fall asleep. This system can work for us sometimes. But our seven-year-old can get very scared in the night. So one of us typically lies down on the floor of the room he shares with his brother and spends a few minutes just being there.

In our house, although the plan does vary slightly from day to day, my husband generally washes the dinner dishes, then takes a few minutes to himself to glance at the newspaper. After washing-up time he comes upstairs to read to our seven-year-old while I read to the four-year-old. After book time, while I'm singing the couple of songs I sing every night to each child, my husband is prone on our bed, waiting in the wings. Then he is called in for his turn. He enters the room warming up his voice with a couple of deliberately silly operatic vocalizings before singing his two signature songs—"Corinna, Corinna" and a bedtime scat tune of his own invention. Then he takes his place on his back in the middle of their floor.

We settled on this system because when the children were very young—nursing, toddling, demanding, needing me in the middle of the night to nurse or comfort them, requiring all of my attention every waking hour—I was never very good at spending time with them once I felt bedtime had been reached. I'd get extremely short-tempered and would feel pushed to my limit. But my husband, who's at work all day, was happy to have an excuse to pass out on the floor somewhere, anywhere. Now I get enough sleep, and have time to myself in the mornings and evenings. These days, lying on the floor in the dark doesn't bother me. I like letting my body settle into the floor and my mind wander aimlessly. If I really need to, I use the time to plan my work for the evening. Sometimes I bring in a flashlight and read for a while.

Still, my husband's the principal floor presence, and I use the next minutes to visit my ten-year-old in her room, where she's now reading in bed. Sometimes she wants to chat about things. Other nights she wants to be left alone with her book and her thoughts. Sometimes she wants me to turn off the light right away so she can go to sleep. Other times she's not completely ready to sleep, and I leave her reading in bed with the light on. She's old enough now to be comfortable turning off her own light. And because she's in bed so early, there is no pressure on her to fall asleep right away. What the experts call her "sleep onset delay" can be adjusted, depending on her mental and physical state. All she needs is those ten-odd hours; she's got time on either end of the night.

I know one mother who spends a half hour visiting each of her three children on their beds before they go to sleep. She begins with the five-year-old at seven, then moves to the eight-year-old at seven-thirty, and winds up with her eldest at eight. Those waiting their turn read in bed or lie quietly while they wait. Sometimes my friend falls asleep while lying with her youngest, and the two older children put themselves to bed.

There are indeed many ways you can put your children, and the parenting day, to bed. Play around with variations that work for you and your children. Bring your own wisdom to bear on what everyone in your family needs in order to go to sleep feeling good, but acknowledge that even at its best, a happy bedtime will not guarantee that everyone in the family will feel all's right with the world. No matter what you do, some children will be filled with a nameless dread at the end of the day. The end of the day is, after all, the death of the day, and for some sensitive children, nothing you can say or do will overcome the suggestiveness of the darkness at day's end.

Throughout human history, darkness, sleep, and night have assumed mythological, archetypal significance. In *The Promise of Sleep* William C. Dement reflects on some of this metaphorical baggage:

Night itself was, and is, otherworldly, rubbing up against the unknown, close kin to death. An ancient concept with enduring influence was the idea that sleep is a short death, and death is a long sleep. In ancient Greece, Hypnos, the god of sleep—from which we get the word hypnotism—and Thanatos, the god of death, were believed to be the twin off-spring of the night. Sometimes small figurines depict them as young babies, each one suckling on a breast of Mother Night.

In the final analysis, consider bedtime well served if, at worst, you instill in your children a feeling of resignation and acceptance that it has to happen no matter what, at the particular time you say each and every day.

Once I leave the room at seven o'clock, I do not expect instant sleep unless they are unbelievably worn out from the day. And even then, as Marc Weissbluth theorizes, extreme fatigue in babies and young children can manifest itself as extreme wiredness, and their sleep will not come easily. Because I honored the nap all through their early childhood, my children seldom went to bed hypertired and wired. They went to bed just before the wave of sleepiness would carry them off.

When my youngest child was still napping and his brother was in kindergarten, the three-year-old used to be ready for bed at seven but not ready for sleep. My six-year-old, on the other hand, could barely function after six-thirty. No matter. The youngest, whose good sleep habits were formed when he was six weeks old, is accustomed to a lights-out self-soothing time. Often I hear him talking quietly to his stuffed animals. This kind of noise does not keep his brother awake, and perhaps even soothes him to sleep. When the four-year-old is ready he goes to sleep too.

As for our ten-year-old, she is old enough to understand why we do what we do, and old enough (and sensible enough) not to feel the words *you seem sleepy tonight* to be an allegation she must disprove. For years I fell into the same trap whenever my children were tired. Watching their behavior deteriorate, I would always comment, "You are so tired." I couldn't help myself. The words just came out. But by saying this I inevitably provoked an explosion of rage. "I'm not tired!" they'd scream at me, throwing themselves further over the edge. I always regretted these remarks of mine, but never seemed to be able to censor myself before uttering them. It was as if I had to excuse their behavior somehow, find some rational explanation for it, or else be overwhelmed by the display.

Then one day my son, then about six, rounded on me after I'd declared how tired he was. "You know, a person can be crabby and not be tired!" he fumed. Of course he was right. If I see unacceptable behavior when they are rested and well fed, then I suspect other causes. But I also know my kids, and when they are extremely crabby, generally it is because they are tired. So the practical lesson I drew from this encounter was rather simple: You may think your children are tired, they may very well be tired, but don't tell them or anyone else within earshot that they are tired. Keep it to yourself and get them to bed pronto. Ever since that revelation, I hear parents all the time falling into my old trap of chalking up any kind of unwanted behavior to fatigue.

"Poor girl," says the mother when her four-year-old daughter has tossed a bowl of fruit over her shoulder onto the restaurant floor. "You are so tired."

"I'm not tired!!"

"No, no. Of course you're not tired," the mother replies, rolling her eyes at nobody but herself as she picks up the slimy banana slices.

Given my sorry history on this matter, you can imagine my relief when my daughter finally started saying things like, "I want to go to bed early tonight. I'm really tired."

At any rate, after her good nights with her father and me, she is free to turn off her light when she's ready, that moment or a little later. Recently I asked her about what sleep researchers refer to as *sleep onset delay.*

Me: Once your light's off, how long does it take you to fall asleep?

My daughter: Sometimes it's three minutes, sometimes five minutes, sometimes fifteen minutes, once in a while an hour.

The other night, for the sake of faithful reporting, I lay down on her floor until she fell asleep. Within seven minutes her breathing was regular, and she did not stir as I left the room. This experiment was immaterial, though. Because her bedtime is seven o'clock, it doesn't really matter to me how long it takes my daughter to fall asleep. Sleep onset can be up to an hour if she's got something on her mind, or instantaneous if she's exhausted. With twelve hours at her disposal, and only ten or ten and a half of those needed for sleep, she has room in her schedule for different states of mind.

Sometimes I arrive at my desk to get to work and my seven-year-old approaches. He's scared. He can't go to sleep. He keeps thinking scary thoughts. After many years of dealing with this issue with this particular child, and trying countless solutions that may have worked once or twice but ultimately failed (including losing control and getting angry), I finally stumbled upon something that has seemed to work for the last year. Brace yourself because it's kind of crazy: I give him the shirt off my back. I peel off the turtleneck or T-shirt or sweater and offer him the body-warm garment to sleep with. Luckily my desk is two inches from my closet, so I make the change out of his view in my closet and get myself into something else right away. Who knows what exactly makes this gesture so resonant? It could be the smile with which I take the action, a smile that he picks up and returns to me because it signals that all is well between us, even though he's crossed his threshold after seven o'clock. It could be the fact that I am so obviously giving him something so close to me. It could be that lying in bed holding and breathing in the aroma of his mother is unbelievably soothing. All I know is that it works every time. Satisfied and content, he patters back to his bed or to ours (I don't care which) and settles down to sleep.

I try not to think about the moment when, all grown up, he's lying on the couch and the therapist asks him about his daily life as a child.

"Well," he'll say thoughtfully, "I often had trouble going to sleep, and my mother would strip off her top and give me her shirt to sleep with. Then I could fall asleep."

"I see," says the shrink. "And how did you feel seeing your mother do this?"

A word or two about the midnight hours. I care very much that my children are tucked into bed around seven o'clock. I do not care if, in the middle of the night, they crawl into our bed. This doesn't wake up me or my husband, and is most often due to one of them having a bad dream. Especially regarding the seven-year-old, who has always been plagued by nightmares, I am not ready to ban the practice. I have nothing against the idea of the family bed; I am concerned only that we all get enough good sleep. To the extent that he is wandering out of habit and not fear, I'd like this pattern to change. Recently we rearranged the twin beds in the boys' room into bunks, and our older son now sleeps in the top bunk. So far, this change alone has been holding him in place all through the night. We'll see. In a way I'll be sorry to see this phase end, and in a way I won't.

•   •   •

At this point I can imagine a reader saying, "All of this sounds reasonable on paper, but how in the world can I make my real live children go to bed earlier? They've had no real routine for years.

Or, they've had a routine, but it ends at nine-thirty or ten. How do I even begin to establish a new schedule with them?"

As I mentioned earlier, it's easier to prevent bad habits than to correct them. Setting up your family's routine is much easier to do when the children are babies. But let's say you have preadolescent children—ages five, seven, nine, whatever—who might be resistant to change. They know what's what and will be suspicious of your suddenly trying to pull a fast one.

Answer: Don't pull a fast one.

When your teeth are crooked, you visit an orthodontist. She doesn't yank out your cuspids and reroot them in the correct positions. She fits you with pieces of metal, plastic, and rubber that firmly but incrementally push your teeth where they need to be. Braces are merely guides; straightening teeth takes time. Likewise with your bedtime schedule. Shifting your schedule to an earlier one will not happen overnight. Gentle, incremental change over time will result in the bedtime of your choosing. Both the age of your children and the hour at which they go to bed right now will determine how long it will take to adjust.

If the 7 o'clock bedtime appeals to you, you can have every hope of putting it into practice. Here's how.

For a child between fourteen months and four years old, you have a lot of variables to play with. This child has no sense of clock time and relies upon you to structure her day. Your first duty is to figure out what the ideal schedule would be, both for your family and for your child. Does she need a total of fourteen hours of sleep in every twenty-four-hour cycle? Thirteen? Figure out how much of her total sleep needs are met overnight, and how long she needs to nap in order to make up the remainder of this total. (Seek professional help here, if necessary.) If she's been going to bed at eight-thirty, begin by putting her to bed tonight at eight-fifteen. (Remember that dinner will have to be served no later than six-fifteen. Review the schedule in order to pace the afternoon.)

The next morning, notice what time she wakes up, and think

about nap time as having to happen fifteen minutes earlier than usual. What do you need to do to make sure your child will be ready for lunch and a nap a little earlier than usual? Fresh air and physical play usually do the trick. Work the two bedtimes— midday and evening—earlier and earlier in fifteen-minute increments until you reach seven o'clock. Expect setbacks and frustration, but stick with it. And remember that it's easier to make the shift now than later on in your child's life, when he begins to tell time.

Children between ages four and eight have usually grown out of their nap but don't yet live by the clock. Book time is book time; it's not necessarily seven or six-thirty or six. You and you alone are responsible for making the fifteen-minute shifts. This means that you can make the changes you need to make without calling too much attention to the day-to-day alterations. After a few days you will wind up at the bedtime of your choice without any explaining. Morning awakenings ought to adjust after a day or two to the new routine, but this may take time. Be sure to use blackout shades to help with sunlight in the spring and summer. Also be sure to sustain the rhythm through the weekends, at least until the patterns are set.

Be prepared for some raw nerves until your child's sleep/wake cycle adjusts to the change and he's getting his full complement of sleep. If you are questioned, feel free to explain to a child of this age why you are doing what you are doing. You could say something like "I'm trying to help you get a better night's sleep so that you'll feel better during the day. I have learned something I didn't know about sleep and I'd like to use what I know to help you."

I've experienced many instances of having to change a long-standing policy with respect to my children. It takes nothing away from your authority to admit to wrongheadedness. People make mistakes, and sensible people learn from their mistakes. Even parents. Ideas and beliefs can change over time; when you admit the need for change you are modeling flexibility of thought, something you want to cultivate in your children.

Children between nine and puberty will be more set in their ways and are likely to have habits long indulged by well-meaning parents. To get children of this age to bed earlier, you may have to think about changing some of your rules regarding television and computer time. You may have to adjust your extracurricular activities. You may, in fact, have to rethink your whole way of life. (I elaborate in chapter 4 on strategies for accomplishing this.) Children in this age group are increasingly targeted as independent, power-wielding consumers of culture, of clothing, of toys and games, and of food. They are reported to spend fourteen billion dollars a year in the marketplace. For you as a parent to come between your preteen and the free-for-all of the open market is not easy, but it is essential if you want to put them to bed at a reasonable hour. Ten-year-olds have no business at the mall on a Saturday night.

Once you've decided that an early bedtime might work for your family, announce to your kids that you'll all be trying something new. As with the younger children, start out slowly by serving dinner two hours before the new bedtime on Day 1. If your nine-year-old has been going to sleep at nine-thirty, aim for nine-fifteen and eat at seven-fifteen. Make the days rich and full, and let your children know that the healthy thing to do when they're tired is to go to bed. Keep at it. Talk to them. Encourage them when they've had a good night's sleep. Seek help and support from the sleep specialists in your community, from schoolteachers and administrators. And remember that no matter how sassy and savvy a prepubescent child may sound, he's still very much a child. You can do what's right for him in spite of his protests.

Extenuating Circumstances:
Coping with
Exceptional Nights

Systems ought to be judged by their ability to withstand the most challenging conditions. Show me a fancy knot that comes undone when you're dangling by it from a cliff and I'll say, righteously, "That was no kind of knot." But show me a simple slip knot that can hold while a refrigerator is being lowered three stories and I'll say, "Now that's what I call a knot."

Likewise with the 7 o'clock bedtime. It is a useful system for running your day-to-day life during the school year. It makes for a peaceful, predictable feeling in your home, and cradles your children in its embrace. But what happens when life throws curveballs? What happens when you want to take a trip? Or when someone in the family falls ill? Or when Aunt Myrtle comes to visit for three weeks because Uncle Gene has died and she is lonesome for family? Or when you are just plain exhausted and more than anything want to go out to dinner with your husband?

At these times you will begin to appreciate the ancillary rewards of sticking to the schedule. The 7 o'clock bedtime helps you swing through all kinds of curveballs, and if nothing else, the marveling it will elicit as onlookers witness your routine will flatter your vanity.

Let's look at some of the extenuating circumstances—travel, illness, special evening events, house guests, and going out on a date—that will challenge the system to prove its worth to you and your family.

Travel

One of the gifts of travel is the opportunity it provides to leave routine behind. Traveling with children ought to mean, to one degree or another, that we relinquish our hold on routine, or that we allow the routine to relinquish its control over us.

On the other hand, trips can be very trying experiences for children, who are usually extremely protective of the world as they know it. New faces, new places, and new experiences may dazzle and stimulate kids, but all of this newness can also create a great deal of anxiety for them. It's not a sign of inflexibility; it's perfectly normal. Which is why parents often see their children behaving in atypically uncooperative ways while on vacation. Uncomfortable feelings will make children behave in unacceptable ways. This is how they cope with change.

For this reason, it is important that you be aware of the effect travel can have on your particular child. Babies will experience trips in one way, toddlers in another. Preschoolers and school-children go on vacation in their own ways. You will have to judge for yourself how much of the bedtime routine you take along with you and how much you leave behind.

Your decision will depend on several factors:

- The length of the trip. If it's just a weekend, it may be worthwhile to bag the schedule altogether just to see what happens. If the excursion is four or five days or longer, your interest may be served best by sticking to the schedule, even if it's modified by thirty minutes or so.

- Whether you will be changing time zones. Reckon bedtimes as follows: Travel an hour to the east and your kids will go to bed at eight instead of seven. An hour to the west and you may have to put your kids to bed at six. A three-hour change or more will be more disruptive. Go with the flow for a few days before establishing a schedule in the new time zone.

- Where you will be staying. If you're in a hotel, are you prepared to stay in the room with your child while the older kids and adults eat out? If you're staying with friends or family, is it important to you not to disrupt the schedule in your host's home? Or is it worth it to you to keep your child balanced and agreeable during the trip by ensuring he gets enough sleep? This may mean feeding young ones separately. Will this be possible?

The truth is that if you really want to, it is possible to stick to your schedule whether or not you're at home. However, even if the actual hour is totally abandoned, try to stick to the routine. That is, bring the books and read them. Sing the songs. Tell the stories. You can cut all of this shorter, but your children will really appreciate the effort you make to keep their bedtime—wherever the bed at whatever the time—something they can count on.

When our daughter was six weeks old we took her by car from Baltimore to New York City for a mid-December family event. Packed into our Honda Civic hatchback with clothes, car seat, diapers, and the various accoutrements of infancy, I felt like a Victorian matriarch presiding from the passenger seat, chatting

with my husband and glancing back every two minutes to make
sure the baby's head was not tipped forward onto her chest,
thereby cutting off her air supply. Here we were, a family, on the
road. How flexible and adventuresome it all seemed! Finally I felt
like the proud mother I was hoping to project. Driving along the
Jersey Turnpike I felt myself laughing in the carefree way I had
before the effects of parenthood took hold some eleven months
before. For the first time in ages I felt like myself, not like the
tautly strung, highly distracted wire of anxiety I had become
since the overwhelming sense of responsibility settled on my
spirit. As things turned out, that car ride was the high point of the
weekend.

We attended the parties in good faith, passing the baby to only
a small circle of close family, watching her fontanel thump away
as she slept in smoke-filled restaurants in a relative's arms. I
nursed her compulsively, dashing into bathrooms every twenty
minutes or so. Only when I noticed she was perspiring profusely
did I realize that I had dressed her in so many layers (the weather
was extremely cold) that she seemed to be on the brink of heat
stroke. For some reason it had not occurred to me that whatever
the outdoor temperature, indoor climates generally do not fall
below seventeen degrees and hence require multiple layers of
cotton, fleece, and wool. From that point on I worried about de-
hydration, and nursed her even more. In her diaper appeared
some greenish streaky stuff, which worried me too.

At the final party, as she slept in her car seat, which I had
parked under the grand piano in my mother's apartment, I began
to wonder if it had been wise to make the trip. In retrospect, it
seems obvious to me that I was still too new a mother to put
myself in such a social situation with so much kith and kin. I
wasn't quite sure of my tone as a parent, not quite formed enough
as a mother to advocate for myself and my child. I'd get caught
up in a conversation with some adult, and suddenly realize that I
had a baby sleeping under the piano, and what if I hadn't looked

at her for ten minutes? Who would make sure she was okay? What if somebody tried to pick her up? And what was that green stuff in her diaper, anyway? One person said it was the brussels sprouts I'd been eating. Someone else said the baby needed to see a doctor, that smeary green stuff was a sign of gastrointestinal virus. I had been living a myopic existence for six weeks, training my eye on things like the curl of her lip and the tulip-shaped red blotch between her brows, and suddenly I had to focus on the land of the loud giants. The switch was too drastic.

Needless to say, she hardly slept at all the whole time we spent in New York. When we got home, I was a wreck. It took me another month to get my feet steady, and when I braved a second trip up to New York, this time by train and alone with the baby, we were fine. She and I shared a bed at a friend's apartment, and she napped on a couch when she was tired. Those four weeks made us that much more flexible.

Before you hit the road, know yourself as well as your baby. Don't put yourself in a situation with a very young baby if you have any foreboding that the experience will be a difficult one for you. On the other hand, traveling with only one child is comparatively easy. Take advantage of this time when you can. The time may come soon enough when your family will grow and you will not be able to pick up and go just like that.

●   ●   ●

Because we made so many sleep-related mistakes with our first child, I'll mention two more trips on which it became clear that our sleep strategy was failing. When our daughter was seven months old, we drove up to the Adirondacks for the wedding of an old friend. We'd been given our own bedroom in a lovely lakeside cabin, which we were sharing with an elderly female friend of the family. Our daughter could not fall asleep on her own and would not sleep in the Portacrib. She was used to sleeping with us, but would not remain asleep for longer than an hour or two. She would not be comforted by nursing and spent whole chunks of the night crying, tossing, and flailing about. Our cabin mate hinted not at all subtly that we were doing everything all wrong, that if we would just lay her down in that crib she would sleep through the night.

Obviously, the baby needed to be put to sleep with some authority. But such authority we could not muster. We told ourselves that if she were really underrested she would not be as cheerful and alert as she was by day. We told ourselves that our baby was an exception, because at the unbelievably early age of six months she was doing what the baby books called cruising: walking along the floor on her two feet while holding steady with her hands on a couch or some other stable support. Surely such a physically precocious child could not be expected to settle like a blob at sleep times.

On the way home from this trip we stopped off at a dear friend's in New Jersey. Our friend had set up the dreaded Porta-crib. I dreaded it because of the pressure I felt to have my baby perform in it, sleepwise. Our friend then had a four-year-old and a thirteen-month-old. After a toddler/kid dinnertime, our friend put her two children to bed, one with a story, the other with a bottle in a rocking chair. When she came downstairs I was still going through my nursing, laying-baby-down-asleep, baby rousing, renursing, relaying routine. Adult dinner was waiting on me. Finally I got her to bed in the crib. An hour or so later she was up and crying, and the rest of the evening was shot to pieces. My friend said I ought to consider doing things a little differently. Still, I wasn't ready to.

The very last trip we took with our daughter before finally arriving at the breaking point was to Europe when she was almost ten months old. Our destinations were Copenhagen and Berlin. We flew to Copenhagen first to visit my husband's brother and his family. The plane ride was fine. And even the time change was no big deal, except for that first night, which I recall as one long torture session. Once we settled in for the trip, which would end in Berlin at my sister's wedding, the only real problem we had was the same problem we had at home: getting the baby to settle down and go to sleep for long stretches on her own. By now our daughter was walking all over the place. Watchful, physically active, alert, and happy—she never seemed to us the profile of a sleep-deprived child.

Of course, my husband and I exhibited every single one of the characteristics of sleep-deprived parents: We were hypersensitive, defensive, scatterbrained, ill-humored, and beyond tired. In those days I would regard strangers on planes, buses, and grocery store lines and think, "Look how normal she looks! She's smiling and happy. I bet she sleeps through the night. How lucky she is!" I used to think to myself that if only I could sleep more than two or three hours at a stretch, I would never, ever pity myself for anything ever again.

At any rate, there in Berlin I remember putting the baby to bed with my husband in an apartment upstairs from the wedding party, and joining in the celebration with my whole heart— dancing, smiling, actually enjoying myself. Around two in the morning my husband appeared at the party with our weeping ten-month-old, who had roused and was crying angrily. I excused myself and went off to bed with her in my arms.

On the day of our departure, a small, curvaceous, husky-voiced South American friend of my sister's approached me with a tiny, amber-colored, unlabeled glass bottle containing some sort of potion. It was a sleeping draught, the woman said. I should give it to my daughter just as the plane was taking off and she'd sleep the whole eight hours. Finally, she said knowingly, I might get some rest. I took the bottle in silence. I have to admit it actually crossed my mind to give the potion a try. Somehow, of course, I realized that this was going too far, that if I could spend even a fleeting moment considering administering some mysterious

narcotic to this precious child of mine, then I needed to recon-
sider our whole outlook.

Our plane was delayed; we missed our connection in New York
for Baltimore and had to spend the night at the airport. Our
daughter spent the night sleeping on my back, in the backpack,
as I folded myself forward over my legs so she could lie horizon-
tally.

This was the low point of our sleep history. If this were a book
about fighting to get off alcohol, at this point I'd be unconscious
in the gutter on a rainy night with an empty bottle of Jack
Daniel's loosely clutched in my pale hand.

So we made a resolution: As soon as the baby could utter the
word *mama*, signaling to us by this that she had made a cognitive
separation between herself and me, and hence would not be prematurely yanked from her matrix of comfort and unity, we would
enforce a going-to-sleep routine. In those days Ferber was the
new rage. Yes, we would Ferberize her. Just as soon as we heard
those magic syllables.

What a crackpot of theories I was! If there was a theory that
appealed to me, I stuck to it fanatically. Cognitive separation?
Matrix of unity? Boiled down to their essence, all of my cocka-
mamy notions originated from the same motive: I simply could
not bear to let my child cry herself to sleep. And why not? No
surprise here: As a young girl, I had done quite a bit of crying
myself to sleep, albeit for entirely different reasons. Consequently,
I had trouble distinguishing one kind of cry from another. Any
cry was a cry for me. When I heard my baby cry, only one thing
made any sense at all: help her to stop crying. Attach her to my
body and let her suckle herself into oblivion.

I treasured the image of the happy African mother/vegetable
tender whose baby was swaddled against her body all day and
all night. This mother was so familiar with her baby's cycles
she'd simply hold him out from the sling every few hours and let
him urinate and defecate on the earth beside her feet. That was

my ideal. Unfortunately, I was not a tuber-tending African mother dwelling in a cozy hut with supportive villagers a mere ululation away. No. I was a part-time newspaper reporter living in a Baltimore row house, wedded to a graduate student who spent his days and nights tearing his hair over Wordsworth's *Ode: Intimations of Immortality.* Our brisk, Teutonic, no-nonsense, ever-sweeping next-door neighbor, whom we affectionately called The Widder Mary, was a far cry from the loving gentle extended-family mother figure I knew from my anthropology books. Beginning when our baby turned six months old, The Widder Mary started asking me when I intended to "break her to the pot."

Really, all of this was a shame. The traveling I did with our first child that first year only brought into sharper focus all the things we were doing wrong. Had I known better, had I given her half a chance to establish control over her own falling asleep, I might have had a bunch of nice trips with my baby. As it was, I had a bunch of intense away-from-home experiences with her as an infant, some of which were nice, but all of which bore the cross of extreme sleep deprivation and nighttime frustration. To those of you starting out with baby number one, I encourage you to establish the kind of routine that allows you to get the rest you need. In this instance only, try to do as I say, and not as I did.

●   ●   ●

A quick bit of reassurance: unbelievably, our daughter's sleep straightened out incredibly quickly once we took the reins firmly in hand when she was fourteen months old, and she appears to have suffered no lasting damage from that first year of shattered nights. The lesson, to me, seems clear: Recognize when you are miserable (or, in my case, out of your mind) and do something about it. You're going to make mistakes whatever you do. Kids are resilient and forgiving. Don't let yourself get so exhausted that you can't enjoy those months. Becoming fully responsible for another person is hard enough without compounding the degree of difficulty by sleep deprivation.

That said, given my outlook at the time, there is no way I could have done anything differently in those days; I treasured those long nights of sleeping beside a sleeping baby, and the long afternoons reading in an easy chair, holding her as she napped for hours. I cannot honestly say I regret what we did, and I know that if I were starting tomorrow as a young mother with a new baby, I would probably make all the same decisions. That was my life then, and I lived it entirely in the present; it's only in the retelling that it seems so exquisitely, impossibly ridiculous. But one thing was certain even then: I could not raise my second and third child under the same system.

●　●　●

If your family includes an infant and a preschooler, traveling is a logistical challenge. But if the plans are well laid, the trip will be a success.

To preserve as much as possible of your routine, try to book your flights or plan your long drives to coincide with naptime. (If it's economically feasible, try to book all flights direct and non-stop to your destination.) If you've got a baby between six and fifteen months old taking two naps a day, try to fly during the morning nap. If you arrive at lunchtime, you can eat and put your preschooler down for a nap at her regular time, around one or two. Sometime while the older child is asleep, you can put the baby down for his second nap. Lo and behold, you're on schedule for the 7 o'clock bedtime.

Bear in mind that while life with children, and especially traveling with children, is never predictable, you will never regret the attempt to make things work out just right. If the flight or drive is especially long, carry along snacks and meals that you can offer at the accustomed time. Give regularity a fair shot, and you may be surprised at how settled your children can be. The amazing thing is how a schedule can help you adapt to all kinds of bizarre life twists.

When our son was three months old, we brought him and our daughter, then nearly three, to New York, for yet another family wedding. This baby was a happy thumb sucker; I could lay him down awake atop his special blanket on the floor of an airplane and watch him suck himself to sleep. Given our first experience with infancy, it seemed a miracle. At the wedding he made a brief appearance in his fancy little outfit, but around seven I changed him into pajamas and let him fall asleep in a carriage while the rest of us sat at our tables and chatted. There's even a picture of him asleep on his lambskin rug on the landing of the restaurant.

Two months later we returned to New York for Thanksgiving. Just after the holiday we were called away to attend the funeral of my grandfather in Dallas. We were a family of four, but we could move around the country with a respectable amount of flexibility because of the schedule we had internalized. Our daughter napped midday all through the long weekend; our infant found comfort on his lambskin and with his thumb.

During nap times we paid no calls, and the children received no visitors. I have never felt even a smidgen of guilt when keeping my children asleep through visits. Who wants to meet a whining, difficult child? Moreover, who wants to present their offspring in this compromised condition, sheepishly murmuring the lame "he's really tired this morning" to excuse the embarrassing behavior. Sure, people know what kids are like when they're tired. And some people are even sympathetic. But what's the point? I'd choose a pleasant adult conversation concluded by a brief moment with a rested child any day.

With older children—that is, with children who require no

midday naps—traveling is fairly straightforward. Nevertheless, it still seems appropriate to account for their schedules when booking flights or planning drives. Try to leave after breakfast when children are freshest. Try to eat dinner on the first night at close to a normal time. Try to bring whatever special blanket, stuffed animal, or treasure ensures that your child feels comfortable in a strange bed. I usually limit such personal belongings to one or two, and require that the child carry it in his or her plane bag along with whatever small toys, playing cards, or books they've packed for their traveling amusement.

Let's conclude this section on traveling with a vision of the 7 o'clock bedtime miracle in action. When our kids were two, five, and nearly eight, we took them to Sweden for the month of July. We were staying with friends in their family's five-bedroom house on a beautiful island in the Gulf of Bothnia. The sun set around midnight and rose by two or three in the morning. Our two older children shared a room. Our two-year-old slept in a Portacrib in his own room. My husband and I shared a third room. We were all downstairs. Our friends occupied two bedrooms upstairs. Here's how it worked: At five-thirty, after long days of playing on the beach, canoeing, sailing, playing in the playhouse and on the seesaw, gamboling among the wild strawberries, and hiking, one adult fed dinner to all five children. While one or two grown-ups prepared the adult dinner, I or my husband washed our children, read to them, sang to them, and pulling the shades down against a fully sunlit sky, put them to bed. We elder folk then had four or five hours of evening to ourselves, often concluding with a bedtime visit to the sauna around ten-thirty and followed by a cooling off splash in the bay. In the land of the midnight sun, the 7 o'clock bedtime reigned supreme. I rest my case.

Illness

Sleep is the best medicine.

A sick child needs to sleep just as a well child needs to play.

An ill child needs to feel safe and comforted.

Every decision you make regarding your ill child ought to be made with these truths in mind. Schedules, routines, and formulas may be suspended when your child is ill. Does she feel better in your bed? Do you sleep better with her next to you so you can check her temperature with your lips all through the night? Fine. Put her to bed in your bed. Is your spouse disturbed by the midnight action of a sick house? Fine. Sleep in the child's bed or on the floor of his room. Or send the spouse into another bed somewhere so you and the sick one can be alone.

Would she nap if she were bundled in a chair downstairs instead of isolated in a bedroom? Fine. Bundle her downstairs. Is the baby fretful and wakeful unless she's in your arms? Fine. Quit the housework. Quit talking on the phone. Get a bunch of magazines and books and sit in a chair all day holding her in your arms. Fall asleep yourself if you need to. Believe me, you'll look back on this day with nothing but fond nostalgia.

Nothing supersedes the goal of getting your child well again. It may be difficult to return to the schedule, but until that moment, do whatever you need to do to bring her back to health. To an older recovered child complaining of the cessation of indulgence, you simply say, "That's the way we do it when you're sick. Now you're all better and it's better for you to go to bed the regular way."

Of course, there are those gray zones of illness that are more difficult to read. A simple head cold really doesn't call for the kind of suspension of routine required by the flu, or bronchitis, or chicken pox. And actually, even if your child seems to you to be quite ill, follow his lead when it comes to bedtime routines. If he takes comfort in following the evening ritual, if he doesn't seem to require any special treatment, stick to routine. The goal is to see the child sleeping off the illness. Don't feel that because he is ill you absolutely must be by his side at all times. Some children actually prefer to be alone in a darkened room when they're sick, and they recover better when you are nowhere to be seen. Keep a monitor on in the room or give the child a bell or whistle so he can get your attention if necessary, but there is nothing wrong with going about your business in the meantime.

Here also is another circumstance in which I have avoided using the television. We all grew up associating staying home sick in bed with watching hours and hours of games shows, cartoons, sitcoms, and soap operas. I know that the television kept me awake during hours I would have been better off napping. But it was truly impossible to turn it off. There was always some show I liked coming on in the next hour or half hour, and it just didn't seem worth it to turn off the TV for that interlude. Also, there was something that happened to my eyes and brain during those sick days of marathon TV-watching: I couldn't have fallen asleep even if I wanted to. I became restless and irritable, and napping was impossible.

There are ways to compromise, of course, if you have an ill child over four or five. If she has spent the whole day in bed, either being read to or playing quietly with animals or listening to music or a book on tape; if she has napped once or twice; and if you really feel that it is in her interest to watch some television, then around three o'clock or so you can sit by her side and watch a half hour of some appropriate show. Any longer than a half hour and a child gets that glazed-over look and usually becomes crabby and difficult. By four or four-thirty a sick child is heading toward the end of the day. At five o'clock serve her dinner and proceed to bedtime as you normally do.

An ill child over six or seven who is sick enough to stay home from school and nap midday may not, however, be able to go to bed at the usual hour of seven. In spite of the extra sleep required to fight the illness, the child may just not be tired enough to warrant the regular bedtime. Take this into account when planning the end of the day. Consider it a gift of time. Read a few extra books. Play a round or two of Boggle or hangman. The evening activity after dinner needs to be quiet and soothing, nothing physical or frustrating. (And actually, this is true of anything your child does after dinnertime, sick or well. Go back and review the appropriate activities for children before bedtime in chapter 2 for extra ideas.)

Try not to defer the bedtime past seven-forty-five or eight. If a child has recovered sufficiently to return to school, he will still need a good night's sleep to cope with the next day. Often children relapse into illness because the sudden onset of their regular routine was just too much to handle with a weakened system. Sometimes this is merely because the child has been sent back to school too soon; but often it results from the late bedtimes consequent to a couple of days of minimal activity. Always remember: Kids have to be ready in mind and body to fall asleep.

I am always amazed at the way daily life is entirely suspended when a child is ill. When our daughter was three months old we brought her to St. Louis to visit my in-laws and extended family. She picked up a cold during the brief trip, and we returned to Baltimore with a sick baby. It was her first illness, and suddenly our lives took a turn for the surreal. My husband ran out to buy a humidifier, which he then sanitized with several rounds of bleaching solution. We turned the thing on, and within an hour or so our tiny row house was entirely filled with a cool fog, making it difficult to see beyond an arm's reach. Next, following a suggestion in some baby book or other, we raised one end of the baby's crib mattress so that her head could drain properly when we laid her down to sleep. During her nap she managed to wriggle toward the opposite end so that by the time she awoke her head was pointing downhill. She repeated this shift with every nap. Finally we gave up and simply took turns holding her sleeping form at the proper inclination, even though the weight of her sleeping head put the holder's arm to sleep. For a few days we spent all of our time wrestling with the bulb syringe, refilling the humidifier tank, and calling the doctor for periodic assurance that she would survive the night. I also worried about the mold counts in the house consequent to the rain forest levels of humidity.

Now, of course, illness does not cause such an uproar. Now that we are oh-so-experienced and generally unflapped by all but the most frightening circumstances, our basic rounds of colds and flu are merely events to manage with as much love, patience, and sense as we can manage.

The two symptoms that wreak the most havoc on sleep are coughing and fever.

Any way you slice it, coughing is a pain in the neck. It rouses the child. It rouses you. It often rouses any siblings sharing a room with the cougher. It also exhausts the patient, so that after a night of coughing she appears far worse than she may be because of fatigue. But you need to be careful with remedies that suppress cough, which often result in a severe bout in the morning. Almost every child who coughs all through the night will require a nap the next day. Both conventional and homespun remedies suggest the same thing for the person with a cough: as many fluids as they can ingest.

Likewise for fever, which unless it is keeping the child awake or is spiking alarmingly high can go without treatment. Although I don't scorn medical intervention when intervention or medication is called for, I do tend to avoid ibuprophen, acetaminophen, antibiotics, and over-the-counter decongestants and cough suppressants when coping with minor viruses. I tell my children what I believe: that fever is their friend and ally in fighting off their illness, that the extra heat their bodies generate is what weakens and kills off the germs. I tell them that a strong, healthy body will run a fever, and that fluids, sleep, and time will make them well again. Salt water nasal sprays also work wonders. But again, if I sense that my child is in the kind of pain or discomfort that absolutely prevents rest and recuperation, then of course I'll dose him with the appropriate drug. The overarching rule of thumb with a sick child is therefore sleep, sleep, and more sleep.

There was only one time I felt betrayed by sleep. One dreary gray February afternoon, our eight-month-old son was heading into his fourth hour of an afternoon nap. By then three-hour naps were not unusual for my children, so I didn't think too much of it. But four hours did seem a little excessive. When I went in to check on him, he was semiawake, making a very quiet sound, and burning hot. He had gone down for a nap with a touch of a runny nose, and he had awoken with a temperature of 104. I whisked him to the doctor, who sent us on to the hospital, where pneumonia was confirmed in one lung. At that point I knew where to draw the line for my kids: over three hours during the day, and something was wrong. It is imperative that you know your own child's cycles, so that you can observe with good judgment any deviations.

Special Events

Your parents are coming to town around the holidays and want to take the whole family—including two children ages four and seven—out to dinner and to see *The Nutcracker Suite*. Matinee tickets are sold out. Your father, who has eaten dinner at six o'clock every night since 1942, cannot sit down to his evening meal before six. Your children are accustomed to eating at five and will be crabby and hungry if dinner is late. What do you do?

This sounds like one of those survival manual questions, where you have to come up with a viable solution ASAP or die in the cold on a frozen mountaintop. Think about what you can come up with on your own to solve this problem before reading on.

Now continue reading to see what I suggest.

If possible, you get your kids to nap using the same routine you use for bedtime. If they are reasonable children, you say that they will enjoy the evening ten times more if they are rested. If they respond well to ultimata and you are prepared to make good on your threat, calmly declare that they cannot go if they do not nap, or at least have a good long rest time.

If your children, knowing what's in store, get so excited about upcoming events that they simply cannot shut down and sleep, then do not tell them about the plans. Happy kids live on a need-to-know basis. They do not really need to be informed in advance. I remember reading the *Little House* books for the first time with my daughter and being absolutely shocked to learn that Laura would awaken one morning and be told that that day was her birthday. But of course it made perfect sense. Birthdays ought to be a surprise. Anticipation of any kind weighs heavily on children, who by their nature live entirely in the present. We see children all the time who are counting the days until Halloween, or until Uncle So-and-So comes to visit, or until a trip to Disney World. This strikes me as an entirely modern phenomenon. Once in a while, it can't hurt to keep them in the dark. Dinner out and the *Nutcracker* can be a surprise you spring on them after nap time.

Still, napping and resting are much easier if their bodies are tuckered out from exertion. If your plan is to put them down for a nap before the big night, you'll have to run them around in the morning so they're entirely exhausted by midafternoon. After a large lunch you initiate the nap-time ritual and give it your best shot. With any luck, you'll have rested children ready to experience a lovely evening out with family.

But let's say your children cannot nap. Let's say that constitutionally they have outgrown the nap and simply cannot manage it. My niece, who is a bundle of life force, falls into this category. She may be tired. Her face may be flushed with fatigue. But when she and her cousins (my children) are told, let's say on a car ride, that they must go to sleep so that they'll have fun when we arrive, the cousins go to sleep and she does not. She cannot. For the sake of this child, who for whatever reason cannot nap, you owe it to your parents to explain that your child is not used to staying up so late and you're not sure how it will work. Probably your parents will say something like, "Oh, now, we used to take you out all the time and you did fine. They'll be fine. Don't be so worried about their bedtime. It's once a year, for heaven's sake."

You'll shrug and hope for the best.

After a late-afternoon rest, feed your children a larger-than-usual snack at three. This snack must last them until six, but remember that you also want them to eat well in the restaurant.

Finally, primped and dressed, off you go. Your kids will probably muddle through just fine, although sometime during dinner you will know in your heart that this isn't going to work because the four-year-old is already starting to melt down. Later in the evening, perhaps when Doctor Drosselmeyer is bandaging up Clara's toy nutcracker, your child's head will bob onto your shoulder. But perhaps not. You never know.

One thing is sure, when you get home around ten-thirty or eleven, prepare for bed under emergency conditions. After administering some late-night succor in the form of cold cereal, move straight to toothbrush and bed. On this kind of a special occasion, forgo the book time. Lights out after tooth brushing. One song, and good night. Then congratulate yourself on a successful evening out with the family.

Of course, just as Sunday morning hangovers followed your Saturday night carousing back in the old days, the day after a special and late night will be a trying one for you and your children. Bloody Marys are out of the question; you must remedy their fatigue in other ways.

If the kids will not nap the day after a special night out, put them to bed at six. To accomplish this, follow the schedule detailed in chapter 2 but serve dinner at four-thirty. If they do nap the next day, they may not be ready for bed at seven, and you may have to set bedtime a little later for just this night. By the second night after the late event, you should be able to stabilize bedtime back at seven o'clock.

Apart from eight o'clock show times, sometimes even a fairly early adult-centered dinner in a restaurant is too much for a child. At two years old, our daughter was considered fairly adept at sitting through a reasonably long meal in a restaurant. Even so, more times than I can recall, my husband would abandon a thick-cut veal chop and clear out to the sidewalk with our screaming two-year-old on his shoulder. You may reasonably inquire as to why it was always my husband who evacuated the toddler. In those days the answer seemed obvious: first and foremost, he always had a soothing way with her (a fact I conveniently reminded him of in these moments). Calming her down was something he did well and with patience. Further, I was the one who still got up in the night if she needed help. I was the one whose adult interaction was limited to goofy confabs with other young mothers weighing the pros and cons of cloth versus plastic and Barney versus Mr. Rogers. I was the one—for better and for worse—whose life was entirely child-centered. My husband left the table because it seemed like the fair thing to do. If we were sitting at a meal with my parents, I did not budge until my plate was cleared. Also, once I declared my precious meal over and we were back home, I would be dealing with the tired, fussy, ready-for-bed toddler while my husband would be leisurely sinking his teeth into that room-temperature chop. Sitting at the table was my way of postponing the inevitable return to routine.

Remember: Any and all changes you make in the schedule will cause a ripplelike reaction in the few bedtimes that follow. You play, you pay.

House Guests

Visitors are always welcome in our house. Having people in the guest room injects new blood into daily life and allows us the opportunity to visit with old friends in an intimate, unrushed way. We like our children to observe that our door is open to the special people in our lives, and that honoring guests is an activity that brings us pleasure.

For the most part, however, I do not change bedtime to suit house guests. If the adults will be eating alone after bedtime, I'll set out hors d'oeuvres and excuse myself to put the kids to bed while my husband and the guest or guests chat. When both of us were required at bedtime—one to manage a baby or toddler and one to handle an older child—we simply excused ourselves for forty-five minutes or so. Everyone we know can appreciate the need for this moment of the day, and comes also to appreciate the peace and quiet of our adult attention focused entirely on them once our children are abed. Guests will typically come up to say good night to the children just before song time. Close friends and family often read an honorary book time, or sing a favorite song, which the children adore.

On the occasions when I plan to eat with the children and our guests, we serve the meal more or less at the children's normal dinnertime. After the main course I may excuse myself from the table as bedtime approaches, then return to the table for dessert and coffee. Of course there are times the children stay at the table for dessert, but only if their behavior is holding up. They know perfectly well when they have lost the privilege of remaining with the adults, and while there may be a fuss, anyone whose behavior is unacceptable is whisked away from the scene.

When making plans for social events like adult dinner parties and meetings, we schedule the gathering for seven or later. If for some reason an affair must begin earlier in the evening, I always try to hire a sitter to manage bedtime so that we can do whatever we have to do to get ourselves ready to host. What our children especially like is to peek downstairs at a dressed-up dinner table and have a brief chance—von Trapp style—to spy on the adults. Sometimes we trot them out for a formal greeting to the company. More often they remain behind the scenes and live their own lives.

One committee that meets in our house is convinced that we have no children at all, so quiet the house is by seven-thirty when the meetings generally start. They accuse us of scattering toys and childish drawings around the house in order to keep up the appearance of having children.

Perhaps I would be more inclined to introduce our children to our company if I did not have terrible memories of being forced to emerge from my bedroom to greet my mother's company. "Just come out and say hello," my mother would say. "That's all you have to do. It's not the end of the world." For me, though, it felt like the end of the world. I hated every second of these presentations. So I suppose, in accordance with the law of equal and opposite reactions, I tend to undertrot my own offspring.

Going Out on a Date

For years my husband and I would not go out until after putting the kids to bed. It was so much easier on the sitter, and we had a better time knowing that the kids were safely tucked away and already asleep before we ever stepped out the door at seven o'clock. And because I always nursed the youngest before bed, I felt committed to that particular bedtime most of all. After all, I thought, the time will come soon enough when we won't have to be here.

Nowadays we can leave whenever we want to. The sitter simply follows my marching orders and the kids are typically in bed within fifteen minutes of their normal bedtime. Naturally, the sitters love the schedule because it makes their job so much easier; they know they'll be able to begin their homework at seven. They like our kids and they know what to expect. The kids enjoy walking the sitters through their routine, proud that they can be the guides of the evening.

*   *   *

It's five o'clock on a Saturday night and the sitter has just arrived. Our children are sitting at the kitchen counter, eating a bowl of pasta dressed with a jar of their favorite tomato sauce. They've got some sliced fruit and glasses of milk. As they eat and chat among themselves, I go over the schedule with the teenager before me. When they've finished eating, I tell her, throw the dishes into the dishwasher. Then you can all go upstairs and wash up, brush teeth, and get into pajamas. The children will have nearly an hour to play (when sitters come they rush through dinner in order to maximize this playtime). Nothing too wild, I plead (a request which is sometimes honored, sometimes not). I tell her to begin book time at six.

Our daughter heads into her room to read on her own or do her own thing. The boys curl up with the sitter and all falls quiet. She reads until six forty-five, then turns lights out and sings and lies down in the dark to settle them down. It is just like every other night, give or take ten or fifteen minutes.

I think one reason this system works so well is that my husband and I do not go out every single Saturday. Because our weekday evenings are all our own, we do not feel the crying, desperate need for rocking weekend nights. So we go out maybe once a month on a Saturday. Maybe. Probably it works out to be less than that. Sometimes midweek we'll go to a movie or dinner, and many Saturdays we plan some special kind of afternoon and early evening with our children (always mindful of the consequences of keeping them up late). Perhaps we'll rent a movie, or go out to dinner as a family, or have a late afternoon ice skating trip in the wintertime.

Still, if we really, really wanted to, or needed to, or if our social lives were such that we had to, we could go out every Saturday night and suffer no ill effects from tired children on Sunday morning.

Incidentally, now that our youngest is well past four years old, on weekends my husband and I allow ourselves the luxury of sleeping in. The boys can help themselves to bread or milk, or their sister can prepare bowls of cold cereal. As often as not, though, they'll just play in their rooms until we rouse and prepare a family breakfast.

Vacation at Home

Now that your children regularly go to sleep during the school week at seven o'clock, what do you plan to do about Fridays and Saturdays? What do you do during winter break and spring break? What do you do during the summer, when the kids are home and the sun doesn't set until eight or nine? Let's look at each case individually.

In our family, Friday night is for collapsing in a heap. The children sense the end of the week as a horse senses a barn after a long ride. My husband lives an active teacher's life and is practically blind with fatigue by Friday afternoon. For these reasons I seldom accept invitations on this night. We observe the Jewish Sabbath, and sit down to a slightly more festive dinner at five or five-fifteen. Breaking from strict observance, I disregard the location of the sun in the sky and light Sabbath candles at our regular dinnertime. At this stage of our lives, a peaceful family moment that allows our children to participate in the ceremony is more important to me than tradition. Someday, perhaps, we will strike the match precisely eighteen minutes before sunset according to the law. But not now. Now we can be off by hours. The bed-time that follows is just like any other night's.

Saturday night, of course, is Saturday night. Whoop it up. This is the night for sleepovers, evening excursions, renting movies as a family, going out to dinner as a family, or splitting off as adults into your own world and leaving the children with a sitter (although as I mentioned earlier, the early bedtime makes mid-week moviegoing and dinners out more feasible, and for us, more desirable). You will need to make adjustments for the children's sleep deficit as detailed in the section on Special Events, but if you are willing to do this, then go ahead and have some fun. Still, at the risk of sounding like a spoilsport, I would recommend that you not put your children to bed later than ten o'clock more than once a month or so. You need to remember what expert Amy Wolfson suggested: Children should not lose or gain more than sixty to ninety minutes of total sleep over the weekend.

Somehow, weekends for many families have become less islands of rest and recuperation and more like sixty hours of an energetic free-for-all of activity. Working parents may feel that they have to catch up on all the time they've not spent with their children during the week. Children's time may fill up with birth-day parties, soccer matches, and math tutoring. Day care providers often say that even without a calendar, they can usually tell Mon-days by the increased fatigue levels of their young charges. It's easier to get the children to nap on Mondays, say these profes-sionals. Conclusion: Before you go all out on a weekend, think about the consequences for your child.

School-year vacations require a different approach. Around the winter holidays, children tend to respond to the increased com-mercial and social frenzy in ways appropriate to their age. Very young children may whine and cry at being bustled from place to place—shopping, paying visits, eating out, staying up late at par-ties. Children under ten may simply run down. Children older than ten may feel a low-level uneasiness concerning all that's expected of them in the company of extended family and friends. Keeping close to your schedule can help offset the effects of holiday overdrive. Try not to mistake wired for happy. Excuse yourself from engagements that seem to be pushing your family too hard.

Last winter break I allowed our children to stay up, lingering around the table with the adults until after ten. I felt like a beatnik—liberated, with-it, unencumbered by bourgeois, dated, middle-class habits and values. Night after night my four-year-old would fall asleep with his head in my lap. His brother passed out on the bed nearby. Our daughter just walked off and got in bed on her own. We adults laughed and talked, absolutely uninvolved in these moments. It was nice for a change.

Well, as you can imagine, the other shoe dropped with a very loud thump not soon after the nightly parties came to an end. The visitors were all gone, and we saw a fair share of disheartening behavior. It took only a few days of normal bedtimes to bring them all around again, but those couple of days were very hard on the children. Were the late, totally unstructured nights worth it? You bet. Just know what you're getting into when you decide to blow off the schedule, and make sure your kids know that they are staying up late because of special occasions, not because things are going to be different from now on.

As for spring vacation, play around as you like within reason. If you want to push bedtime back an hour or so, it can't hurt. If you want to keep things as they are, that's okay too. If the longer hours of daylight keep your kids awake, invest in blackout shades so that seven looks nearly as dark now as it did in December.

Summer vacation is not what it once was: long, seemingly endless stretches of unstructured free time. Most kids go off to full-day camps of one sort or another. If your child has to be up and out of the house in the morning, I suggest holding to a modified version of the schedule throughout the summer. If your child has no scheduled activities that require you to be up and out of the house by a certain time each morning, you need to be the judge of what suits him best. It may be that you can settle on an eight-thirty or nine o'clock bedtime for three months and pick up the earlier schedule as the school year approaches. But it may serve your family's interest to hold bedtime at a firm seven o'clock.

When we dropped off my daughter at a two-week sleep-over camp last summer, I did wonder how she would manage to get enough sleep in such a radically different environment. But breaking from home is breaking from home, and I knew she was up to the challenge in every way. Naturally, after a few nights of eight-thirty and nine o'clock bedtimes, she eventually began to sleep until six-thirty and seven the next morning. The activities of the day were physically demanding, and she simply could not rouse at her usual five-thirty. The cycle shifted on its own, and shifted back when she got home.

Every summer my family and my sister's family gather at my parents' New Jersey shore vacation house. The five cousins typically play outside in the yard from breakfast until noon, when we all go off to the beach for lunch. After lunch they are in the water swimming until five o'clock. Needless to say, after a shower and dinner, they can barely keep their eyes open, and fall into bed like so many raindrops. Only in the last year has my ten-year-old begun to join us for adult dinner at seven, and even she excuses herself to go to bed by seven forty-five or eight. These are truly our halcyon days, which would be anything but if we attempted to keep the younger children up past their bedtime.

4

Facing the

Consequences

I sympathize with the salmon: It's not easy swimming against the current. You can't just flap your fins and pretend the onrushing water doesn't affect your stroke. Establishing a life that incorporates the 7 o'clock bedtime means that you have to draw on all of your personal resources—instinct, strength of character, creativity, and critical intelligence. More specifically, let's look closely at seven particular ways in which you can take an active role in adjusting the general tone of your family's daily life to suit the schedule.

1. Assume the mantle of benign authority with respect to all children, not only your own.

2. Choose with care what you do with your spare time; accept the consequences of saying no to certain activities.

3. Compromise aspects of your domestic management as needed.

4. Ask for help and build a community of mutual support.

5. Create impressive jargon for what you are doing.

6. Severely restrict television and computer games.

7. Communicate regularly with your child's teachers and school administrators in order to keep homework both age appropriate and manageable.

Let's examine these strategies one by one.

1. The Mantle of Authority

One afternoon we brought home one of my seven-year-old's classmates for an after-school play date. We pulled into the driveway and the visitor hopped out of the car. Looking at me, he jerked his thumb toward the backseat and said, "Get my backpack out, wouldja?" At first I thought he was joking and I just looked at him. Then he said, "I said, go get my backpack."

Then I realized that this was the real thing, a real live moment in which utter disrespect and rudeness were being hurled in my direction by a first-grader. So I said, "Listen, Connor, you may not speak to me that way. I don't know how you speak to your teachers or your parents, but you cannot speak to me in that rude and bossy way. While you're with me you have to treat me with respect. If you need help getting your backpack out, ask me in the proper way."

So he did, if begrudgingly, and that was that. My own son threw me a glance, as if to apologize for his friend's behavior, which made the moment even more telling. In that instance, one kid knew right from wrong; the other did not.

Children challenge adult authority in all kinds of ways. In a manner of speaking, that is their job. That's what they need to do in order to see how valid our authority is. Different children are raised to question authority at different ages, and some learn from life experience that adults are often ready and eager to abdicate responsibility whenever they can. Do not be afraid of setting limits and rules on the behavior you expect from your children's peers when they are in your care. There is a big difference between proselytizing your values and demanding respectful speech in your presence. If a playmate comes over and demands something you cannot accommodate, all you have to say is, "In our house, we do such and such. Those are our rules." By respectfully asserting your authority before your children's friends, you are sending two messages: (1) you care enough about the friend's behavior to try to hold it to acceptable, reasonable standards; (2) the rules and limits you establish in your home are to be taken seriously.

Becoming an authority figure is not a matter of turning bossy. Indeed, knowing where to step in and where to back off is yet another element in the art of parenting. In general, think of it this way: When the stakes are low, you let the child have his say. I'm always depressed at the zoo when I see mothers and fathers dragging their kids from animal to animal, as if a visit to the zoo were about seeing the greatest number of creatures in the shortest amount of time.

"Come on, Jasmine. It's time to go see the elephants. Jasmine, come *on*! Don't you want to see the elephants?! Then let's go!"

Poor Jasmine.

When you go out for these kinds of excursions, it doesn't matter if you spend an hour looking at a rabbit who won't move a muscle. As long as you let your child know the consequences ("We can spend all our time here, but then we'll have to visit the bear another day"), it doesn't matter what you see when you go to the zoo. Let your child determine the flow. Show respect for the attention they want to pay to the still-life bunny, and they'll be more likely to respond cooperatively when you ask for their respect later on that night. And if they don't make the connection, then you make it for them: "Remember how I showed respect for our afternoon? Now you have to show respect for our evening."

Another dimension of assuming responsibility is being selective about what you share and communicate with your children. Respect the line between honesty and full disclosure. Children do not really want to know as much as you think they do, or as much as they say they want to know. Potentially hurtful frankness in older kids—"he's just so observant and curious," says the mother when her son asks you why your car is so full of junk—develops in children whose early and natural impulse to question everything has not been seasoned by the instruction to consider the effect of a question on a person's feelings. Some questions are better left unasked, or asked in the privacy of your own home. Try to practice and teach discretion.

Assuming parental responsibility all day long translates directly into bedtime policy, where you are the authority. You will listen to your child and respect his feelings, but you ultimately call the shots. You may make mistakes, but you have the final word. To make your word meaningful, however, try not to use bedtime as either a reward or a punishment. People tend not to "put the child to bed without any supper" in these enlightened days. But I do hear statements like: "If you're very cooperative, I'll let you stay up till eight-thirty tonight." A later bedtime is held out like a carrot, an incentive for praiseworthy behavior. What does such an incentive accomplish? It makes staying awake at night seem better and more desirable than sleeping. It also builds in the child's imagination yet another reason to dislike bedtime. If bedtime were really so great or important, thinks the child, it wouldn't change just because I didn't fight about wearing my new shoes.

Here's another bit of conversation I hear sometimes:

Child: I'm not ready for bed. I want to stay up until nine like Joey.

Parent: When you're eight years old you'll stay up late too. Right now it's bedtime for you.

This is a tricky one. Obviously, and as we've seen, different ages require different amounts of sleep. Still, it doesn't help your cause to advertise again and again that a later bedtime is a function of growing up. We usually think twice before we say to our kids, "When you're grown up you can eat all the candy you want and watch television all day long." Somehow the child knows, though, that even though grown-ups can literally do anything they want, most do not eat candy and watch TV all day. Kids learn from observation that growing up is a matter of stopping yourself from doing what you know is not good. My children are always a little saddened by this realization. As children, they're kept from erring in excess by the vigilance of their parents. As adults, they will be kept from erring in excess by the vigilance of their own consciences. Bottom line: It will never be okay to eat candy and watch TV all day.

To minimize their sense that being older means sleeping less, I try not to call too much attention to the differences in sleep required by the different children in the household. Sleep onset varies from child to child, but there is a general feeling in the house that all the children are going to bed at the same time. Because our daughter has her own room, she has a little more freedom after seven. And as we've seen, I make allowances for the different needs of our boys, who share a room. Sometimes our seven-year-old will read by flashlight once his younger brother has fallen asleep. As I mentioned, the four-year-old is happy chirping quietly while his older brother falls asleep. Acceptance is everything.

2. Use Your Time Well: Learn to Say No

To make the schedule work, you as the parent must choose with care what you do in your own spare time. If you are individually overwhelmed, overscheduled, and overcommitted, you will be unable to create the kind of home environment that enables your children to relax. Create space for yourself so that you can create space for your children.

For more than a decade, I had just about no spare time. Not because I was out conquering the world. Far from it. I took care of my children; I worked part-time. I kept up with the errands and bills, but only barely. I was (and remain) a pretty lousy housekeeper. I read each night for as long as I could stay awake. I was in basic survival mode. There is nothing to be proud of in this fact; I ought to have created some leisure time for myself. Mea culpa.

On the other hand, in the last few years, as the patches of free time have grown, I find that it is a challenge to fill them only with what truly matters to me. When you're filling a bucket that has been empty for a long time you need to pay extra attention to what goes in, in spite of the temptation to throw in anything that catches your eye. Or, another way of looking at the same thing: A vase of flowers in a sparsely furnished room assumes more significance than it would in a parlor full of drapes, furniture, and knickknacks. I've had to learn how to say no.

If you're a gung-ho volunteer, keep your volunteering under control, either during school hours or during the evening hours. I know a jolly, industrious stay-at-home mother who says that if she looks at her datebook and sees a blank square on her calendar then she feels something is wrong. She likes being busy. Even if, like her, you like being busy, try to keep after-school hours and weekends free for your children. See if there's some way you can incorporate your children in your community service. Children can plant trees, collect toys and food for shelters, and read to younger children in day care centers and to elderly people in nursing homes. They can accompany you when you give blood, or work in the garden by your side, even if the garden is simply a pot on a windowsill.

Just as you choose with care what you do as an individual, you must also be extremely selective about what your children do in their spare time. Indeed, the very phrase *spare time* as applied to young children strikes me as fairly dispiriting, suggesting that children are so tightly scheduled that, like adults, they lead lives that can be neatly divided into obligations and leisure. I recall the day our pediatrician, who is considered marvelous because she addresses herself to the patient instead of to the parent, asked my six-year-old daughter what she did in her spare time. My daughter was stumped. I (somewhat cruelly) played along and remained silent to see what she might say. The notion that she, a kindergartner, had spare time was totally foreign to her. Time spared from what? Playing? Eating? Copying out letters at her little desk? Which was the obligation and which the leisure? Every moment of her day carried the same developmental valence. To me, that's what childhood's all about. My daughter paused, and the doctor prompted her with a few suggestions. "Do you watch TV? Do you like to read? Do you . . . ?"

Finally she replied, "I like to play animal games."

Children play because it's fun, but also because this is how they come to terms with life. Even older children, those in the higher elementary grades, require time away from the classroom to sort things out with their peers. My guess is that they learn more about life during the minutes of recess—negotiating games, sorting through conflict, observing their friends, finding a way to move comfortably from group to group, or from solitary to group play—than they do during hours of classroom instruction. Which is not to say that classroom time lacks importance. I'm a big fan of reading and writing and math. I only mean to emphasize the legitimacy and primacy of unstructured playtime. I'm also certain that the critical thinking a child does on the playground is reflected in that child's academic performance.

What does this mean? This means that you might as well save the thousands of dollars you spend on after-school classes and bring your kids to the playground. It means that adults have enough say in the lives of children without dominating every single minute of their time out of school. As any parent knows who tries to extract too much information from a child right after school, most kids are tired of communicating to adults by four. So just be quiet. You're not being uninterested; you're showing respect. If you pay attention, you will soon observe when your child feels like talking.

But what about those legions of gifted and talented kids (have there ever been so many of these before?) who show so much promise in some field or other—whether art, or dance, or music, or athletics—that you feel you are stunting their development if you do not sign them up for this or that extracurricular activity? As I mentioned earlier, one after-school activity a week seems entirely appropriate to me for children up to thirteen or so. Younger children, no matter how much talent you are told they have, or how much you feel they have, do not need structured classes more than once a week to help such gifts flower.

Beyond the weekly classes, a natural-born artist or athlete will find ways to cultivate these gifts unconsciously during free time. Budding Picassos can paint, draw, and play with art materials at home. Future Baryshnikovs can always leap around the house. Innate Einsteins will experiment with water in the sink and drop beanbags from chairs. Latent Mozarts bang pots, tweak stretched rubber bands, jingle keys, and stamp their feet. Embryonic Gretzkys play catch, run, and whack things across the yard with tomato stakes. Natural-born social workers will play pretend games involving complex relations between *Tyrannosaurus rex* and compsognathus. You do not have to treat your children as if they were withered sponges waiting to be dumped in all kinds of classes in order to expand and grow. Just let them play.

"There is nothing that human beings do, know, think, hope, and fear that has not been attempted, experienced, practiced, or at least anticipated in children's play," writes Heidi Britz-Crecelius in *Children at Play*.

A friend says to me about her son, "I think it's important that Ethan [age seven] play soccer because it's good to be on a team." I reply, "Living in a family and going to school are team sports." Any group of people—broadly or narrowly defined—that lives and works for their mutual support and benefit is a team.

One other point seems worth mentioning regarding soccer and other competitive games for young children. Research by the Swiss psychologist Jean Piaget demonstrated that children under the age of six are not even ready to play by extrinsic, externally imposed rules. For young children, all game rules originate from within. This is why I love playing chess, for example, with my four-year-old. It's a free-for-all. Rooks swoop over and across the board to capture pawns. Bishops march directly forward to capture the king, whose loss doesn't affect the game a whit. Pawns sneak between squares and rest on the line between black and white for several turns in a row, then come in and take my queen when I least expect it. Playing traditional games by wholly subjective, ever-morphing rules is a good way to get to know the way your child's mind tends to work.

I've noticed, moreover, that his big sister likes these liberated games, and seeks out her little brother to play chess or the African stone game, mancala, for precisely this reason: Sometimes she likes taking a break from playing by the rules. (Don't we all?) By contrast, our seven-year-old is a more recent arrival in the world of unbreakable rules and has a hard time returning, even temporarily, to playing traditional board games by the seat of his pants.

If, after all of this, you still feel worried about saying no to the busyness of childhood, then do me a favor and talk to your children's teachers. Talk to school administrators. Talk to admissions directors at decent secondary schools and colleges. Talk to psychologists and guidance counselors. Talk to sleep consultants. I'll wager that any one of these professionals will back you up in your effort to scale back the schedules of your kids.

Here's whom you shouldn't talk to: parents forcing their kids onto the fast track as soon as the pregnancy test comes back positive.

3. Make Compromises and Accept the Consequences

People always say, "But you must set your priorities. Get your priorities in order and the rest is easy." Well, it's not so easy. Nothing important is easy. Because there's a flip side to establishing your priorities, and that is having to compromise all the things that fall below first and second place on your list, and accepting the consequences of such compromises.

Cutting back on the things you've been doing with your children in the afternoons and evenings is an example of a compromise you make for the sake of the 7 o'clock bedtime. Other compromises you make for the sake of the rhythm of life are less public. Take housework, that looming, ever menacing, Sisyphean set of activities that never comes to an end. I hate putting things away. I hate straightening up. I hate the constant, unforgiving grind of it. I hate the clutter of papers, bills, magazines, and whatnot that accumulates everywhere I turn. I hate when the drawer knobs fall off and the lightbulbs burn out. But there it is. Housework has to be done, and it is important to communicate to your children that it must be done, and that everyone in the household is responsible for their age-appropriate share of it.

So for the sake of the children and my husband I force myself to keep certain areas manageable. I keep up with all laundry except for my husband's (he takes care of his own), and I try to teach the children to be responsible for their things. On the other hand, I let certain areas of the household go to pot. I can't help it. My closet is a disaster area. As is my desk, and under my desk. Our basement might be considered a fire hazard. I have trouble keeping the smoke alarm batteries up-to-date. I could force myself to be a different kind of person and keep up with all of this, but I do not. I hold my family life and my children dear to me, and if I started catching up with my mess I know that the quality of the hours I have with my family and of my hours alone would deteriorate. I would always rather play I Spy than clear off a counter or change the sheets. When the children aren't around, I'd always rather read a book than sweep. So I compromise the house for the sake of what (conveniently, given my bias) strikes me as more important. Like most people, I have only a certain amount of self-discipline, which I apply to the areas of my life that are important to me. (These areas may shift around, but the discipline is constant.) I face the fact and live with it: I like it when my house is clean and orderly, and the mess will sometimes make me very upset indeed, but housekeeping is low on my list of priorities. For this reason, I am happy to spend a sizable chunk of the money I earn as a freelance writer on freelance housekeepers.

My mother was a perfectly socialized woman of the 1950s, and her daily schedule as a young mother was fairly typical of the period. In the morning, after getting her infant fed, bathed, and changed, she would put the baby (me) in the playpen. There I'd stay for hours while my mother cleaned the whole house, emptied the garbage, did the laundry, and made her morning calls.

When she was all done she'd take me out to the grocery store, or the hairdresser, or to her mother-in-law's for a bridge game. In the afternoons I was fussed over, ogled, and covered with big smoochy kisses by middle-aged bubbes who, my mother says, danced around the room with me in their arms. Then my mother would come home and make a fancy dinner for my father. Somewhere in there I was put to bed with zero fuss.

Today my mother says she regrets the priorities she established. She wishes she had played with me more and let her house go a little. But I know her and I know that she was constitutionally unable to let her household standards fall. Was I happy all those months playing around in my playpen as my mother cleaned and bustled around me? I don't remember. That's not the point. The point is: We are no less socialized than she was. The difference is, today's women were raised to believe that everything is possible, that it is possible to have it all, children, mates, careers, friendships. We believe this even though common sense tells us that this is not possible. We seem to have not absorbed ourselves what we tell our children all the time—"you can't expect to get everything you want." Until parents really understand and accept what it means to compromise (even temporarily) aspects of life that may seem very important—professional ambition, meaningful time with children, romantic moments, a tidy home—setting priorities will have little meaning. Know yourself, and make the compromises you can live with.

4. Ask for Help

Sometimes it is absolutely impossible to stick to the schedule without calling for help. Asking for help is a way of building community, and includes both those desperate cries when things are so bad you cannot go on, and premeditated requests that help you out in the event of a life complication. When people assert that it takes a village to raise a child, they are not claiming that it's okay to neglect your children because there's always someone around—a school, a nanny, a day care center, a neighbor—to pitch in and take over when you give up. Building community, or calling on the village, is about cooperation, about living for a group's collective good.

If you are shut in on a rainy afternoon with two children under four years old and suddenly the emotional temperature of the family is growing too hot—you can't make dinner, you can't even calm the children—it's important to be able to call somebody for help. Maybe the older woman downstairs will let your three-year-old come down and water her plants while you put the toddler in the backpack and cook. Or maybe there's a stay-at-home mother down the street whose child can come over to play and ease the intersibling tension. Seek people whose lives you can connect with for your mutual benefit. The moments we most cherish are the moments when somebody has helped us in a pinch, or when we've bailed somebody else out of trouble.

But asking for help is not always reserved for emergencies. If one of your children has a routine lesson on Wednesday afternoons but you need to be home preparing dinner so that mealtime can happen at five, see if there's someone who can carpool your child home from the lesson. Think of something you can do by way of bartering for this kind of help. Maybe you can double the meal you're preparing so your carpooling partner doesn't have to cook that night. Bartering builds community by assigning value to things and activities that are not simply merchandise. By removing yourself from the economy of hustle, you establish and validate an economy of life.

Consider the method used by a baby-sitting cooperative that had been established among several young families in Baltimore. Their system was fairly simple. Each person started off with a certain number of toothpicks. When you asked someone in the group to baby-sit for you, you paid them one toothpick. Over time, of course, you were supposed to pay out as many toothpicks as you collected. These couples, whose only goal at first was to save money on hiring baby-sitters, wound up building a network of friends whom they (and their children) considered their community.

One other way of asking for help and building community is to turn into an advocate for sleep. Sleep specialists are generally frustrated by the lack of public awareness of sleep as a health issue. Starting in elementary school, children begin learning about the food pyramid. They learn about safe sex and venereal diseases. They learn to wash their hands after using the bathroom. They learn about exercise and about drug abuse. They learn about drinking and driving. Generally, however, they do not learn about the importance of sleep. What happens to their minds and bodies when they close their eyes for the night? Why is sleep necessary? What do dreams have to do with waking life? All of this is interesting stuff, educational stuff that is also a matter of health, fitness, and vitality. It is not good for kids to be kept in the dark about sleep. To change the status quo, parents can lobby school administrators to introduce sleep into the health curricula.

Preschool, elementary school, middle school, and high school are all appropriate venues for learning about sleep in age-appropriate ways.

5. Use Your Jargon

Let's say you are sticking to the schedule, but people start telling you that you are depriving your children of important opportunities, that you are sheltering them in such a way as to make them pariahs among their friends and ignoramuses regarding common culture. You don't feel like reading to them from this book, but you feel like impressing them with what you feel is important about what you're doing. Enlist language. Here's how. This idea, by the way, I lifted directly from Mary Griffith's *Homeschooling Handbook*.

"You can redefine your entire life as educational experiences," Griffith writes. "Going out to play can be socializational development and physical education, grocery shopping becomes consumer math and nutrition education, completing household chores develops concentration and time-on-task skills, and library trips are research instruction and resource identification.

"Translating everyday activities into education jargon can also be reassuring to unschooling parents who worry that their children are 'doing nothing.' Putting life into educational terminology makes it obvious that they are doing a great deal and that we are just not good at recognizing learning that takes place outside the classroom."

6. Avoid Television and Computer Games

Just as you can invest the daily life of your child with unappreciated significance when you put it into highfalutin language, you can really see the intent and meaning of television watching and computer play when you ratchet up the descriptions of these activities.

You may like to think your kid is "just vegging out in front of the TV after a long day at school." That really doesn't even sound so bad. After all, you make dinner, the house is quiet, the kids aren't fighting, you can even talk on the phone as you cook. But here's what science has to say about this moment:

Three effects on learning abilities, all related to attention, have been suggested: 1. some television and videotape programming artificially manipulate the brain into paying attention by violating certain of its natural defenses with frequent visual and auditory changes (known as saliency); 2. television induces neural passivity and reduces "stick-to-itiveness"; 3. television may have a hypnotic, and possibly neurologically addictive, effect on the brain by changing the frequency of its electrical impulses in ways that block active mental processing.

These are the words of Jane M. Healy, Ph.D., in her book *Endangered Minds*. Suddenly, vegging out sounds kind of—well, bad. It's a lot easier saying no to something that you think is bad than to something about which you are indifferent.

Healy also writes, "I am willing to make the leap and suggest, by inducing our children to habituate their brains to too much easy video pleasure, we may truly risk weakening their mental abilities."

Since I've had children, I have come to regard the act of watching television as a narcotic. As an adult I can distinguish good content from bad content, and at times even enjoy applying a critical reader's eye to the programs I see on TV. For my kids, however, I'm convinced that the act of watching is the drug: the medium is the medication. So when I allow my children to watch, whatever it is I am allowing them to watch, I imagine that I am dosing them with something more akin to acetaminophen than to a bit of culture. The younger they are, the less able they are to process the content, and the stronger the effect of the drug.

That television watching is essentially an anesthetizing narcotic was made absolutely plain to me one morning when my daughter had to go to the hospital for minor outpatient surgery. She was having a large freckle removed from her scalp. She was five years old, and the surgeon had not wanted to operate on her because she was so young. He thought she'd squiggle as he worked. After all, he would be injecting an anesthetic into her scalp and then slicing away on the top of her head while she sat there wide awake. I wanted the surgery done and explained to him that I thought she'd be fine. I knew she could sit.

Well, even I was astonished by what happened. There I was, braced to hold her hand and keep her calm. But she had no need of me. A giant television was on in the operating room, and once she had glued her eyes to that dancing bear on the screen, the surgeon could have removed all of her hair and both ears and she'd never have noticed.

Television's disarming ability to remove the viewer's awareness from his own bodily and mental presence, its tendency to so absorb and numb the viewer's attention, to distract the senses from any kind of pain or suffering, makes it comparable to the most powerful analgesics.

In his book *Boxed In: The Culture of TV,* Mark Crispin Miller describes the process by which television alters the mind of the viewer: "No contrast [from commercial to news], however violent, could jolt TV's overseasoned audience, for whom discontinuity, disjointedness, are themselves the norm; a spectacle that no stark images could shatter, because it comes already shattered. TV ceaselessly disrupts itself, not only through the sheer multiplicity of its offerings in the age of satellite and cable, but as a strategy to keep the viewer semihypnotized."

Let Jane Healy give you even more confidence about turning off the boob tube. She writes:

The overall effects of television viewing and other forms of video on the growing brain are poorly understood, but research strongly indicates that it has the potential to affect both the brain itself and related learning abilities. Abilities to sustain attention independently, stick to problems actively, listen intelligently, read with understanding, and use language effectively may be particularly at risk. No one knows how much exposure is necessary to make a difference. Likewise, no information is available about the overall effects on intelligence of large amounts of time taken from

physical exercise, social or independent play, pleasure reading, sustained conversation, or roaming quietly about in
one's own imagination.

It's this last bit that I really want you to hear. Even if TV were a
great thing, and not a narcotic whose commercial content most
often treats your children like pathetic mercenary consumers,
watching it still takes time away from the activities that really
matter to them, and renders them less and less capable of enter-
taining themselves.

A few weeks ago I was down and out with the flu on a Saturday
morning. My husband needed to get his winter grades in and had
to spend the morning at school. I felt horrible and had farmed out
our older children to friends. My four-year-old was home, but I
explained to him that I simply could not get out of bed, that I was
sick and needed to rest. As I lay in bed staring out the window,
wondering if my flu was going to worsen into pneumonia, my son
played on his own from six-thirty until noon, when my husband
came home. During those hours he looked at books. He talked to
his animals. He played long, complicated pretend games. He
came over and sat beside me from time to time. Actually, I'm
not sure what all he did. I was too sick to pay much attention.
Some of the time I was dozing. And the child was absolutely
spent by noon. We proved that five and a half hours of self-
sustaining entertainment must be his limit. Still, I was entirely
amazed.

I love my children and am often dazzled by the resources they
evidence, but I am certain that they are not the only children in
America who can spend their time without television and computers. I assure you that you can get through the day without
television. Trust me, you will get dinner made. You will have some
time to yourself. You may have to do a little bit of parenting, but
certainly, if you have children, then you are prepared to do this.

I have friends who will say, "But some of the most productive, energetic, intelligent people I know are people who spent their whole childhoods watching TV. I know doctors and lawyers and businesspeople, classic type As, who did nothing as children but watch TV. How can it be as bad as you say?" One fortysomething friend takes this logic one step further and remarks, "Look at me. I watched no television at all growing up. I'm the last of a dying breed and I'm a lump, the biggest slouch of all. Not watching TV is no guarantee that your kids won't be slouches."

How can you reply to this argument?

Here we have the destiny offered as a justification (or contraindication, in my friend's case) for the journey. If you really and truly believe that your children will in no way suffer in the long run from spending time on a chair pushing a mouse around and watching shadows play on a screen, or from your allowing the low-level hum of the television to reign for even an hour or two a day in your home, then be my guest. If you buy the message of video-game producers that this stuff is fine, or even beneficial—again, have at it. In both these cases you have more faith than I that these technologies are harmless.

Beyond this, I would bet that my friend who is the self-described slouch has a perfectly rich inner life, an inner reality that lends itself to profound thought, feeling, and creativity. Slouches often have a mental heft that the glittering and bustling type As don't.

In any case, think of my grandfather, who died this winter at ninety-four. Up until his final breath, he was mentally fit and sharp as any adult I know. Every evening for decades he drank a sizable tumbler or two of rye and ginger ale. The idea of performing any kind of exercise struck him as ludicrous. For years he smoked cigarettes and pipes. Did he say, passing his great-grandchildren a jigger of Canadian Club, "Look at me! I smoked and drank for years and am healthy as a horse. Have at it!" Of course not. He surmised quite reasonably that the drinking and smoking that may be acceptable for adults is not at all acceptable for children. Plus, he'd seen enough of his friends die of lung cancer and heart disease to know that he was just lucky.

Regardless of whether juvenile TV viewers and video game players come to good or bad ends, there's a quality of daily life I'm after that is absolutely unserved, relentlessly eroded, by entertainment machinery. Of course we watch television from time to time. We rent movies. It's just not part of daily life, either mine or my children's. Does my fourth-grader feel like an alien among her classmates? Not among those whom she considers her friends, but it does help that her very best friends, twins who attend a different school, are also growing up in a home without a television. The three girls will sometimes compare notes on their experiences in this regard.

One thing my daughter has noticed: When the classroom television and video monitor break down, she is not one of the kids who jump up to lend a hand fixing it. She leaves such tasks to her machine-savvy classmates.

When my children are fully grown, they can decide for themselves how much time they want to spend in front of the television and computer screen. But just as it seems unfair to feed growing bodies candy and potato chips for breakfast, lunch, and dinner, or even (because some people are moderate consumers) for snack every day; and equally unfair to allow them to stay up until eleven every night; it seems unfair to expose for any significant periods of time an immature brain to the flashes and images that emanate from a box. The idea is that having been raised to think, imagine, invent, and accept occasional boredom, my children will, as adults, be in a better position to actively choose with real judgment and discrimination what they want from the culture at hand. In the meantime, they'll continue to sleep through prime time.

With respect to the 7 o'clock bedtime, there's still another giant piece of the TV puzzle we have to slip into place. Apart from the effect TV viewing has on cognitive development, eating habits, physical activity and fitness, aggressive behavior, school performance, and social interaction within the family, scientists have linked watching television with sleep disturbances in children. In 1998, sleep scientist and pediatrician Judith Owens and her research team studied 495 children in kindergarten through fourth grade from three public schools in Portsmouth, Rhode Island. The study, reported in the *George Street Journal*, revealed that "children who watched television just before bedtime had the most difficulty sleeping, resisted going to bed, and woke up most during the night."

Proportionally linked with the sleep disturbances were the number of hours the child watched each day, the amount of television watched close to bedtime, and the existence of a television in the child's own bedroom. Owens wrote in the study:

> There are a number of theoretical ways in which television viewing habits could have this impact on sleep. Television viewing may simply serve to displace sleep time, thus shortening sleep duration to unacceptable limits. The period of time spent by the child in television viewing may substitute for other less sedentary and/or less passive activities (like playing outside, engaging in sports activities), resulting in poor quality sleep. The content of the programs viewed, by virtue of excessively violent and/or stimulating themes, may result in difficulty falling asleep and/or night wakings related to anxiety. The presence of an independent factor, such as poor parental limit setting, may account for both excessive television viewing and bedtime resistance. Finally, parental viewing habits and attitudes about television may impact significantly upon both television viewing habits and sleep in their children.

It seems painfully obvious that watching television in the amounts average American children are said to watch—twenty-five hours a week—should affect their sleep for the worse. I know that there were Saturdays in my childhood, whole days, that I would do nothing but watch television. And I also remember the feeling at the end of those days—dry-eyed, numb, a little dizzy, sort of lonesome, sad, and out of sorts—that accompanied me to bed. I'd lie in bed and wait for sleep, all the while feeling that another day was gone.

7. Keep Homework Manageable

An exercise like any other, the ideal homework assignment accomplishes more than one thing at a time. First, it trains the child to transport material between home and school. Second, it reinforces skills and concepts taught during the school day. Third, it alerts the child's teacher to any problems the student might be having assimilating new concepts or skills. But homework can only accomplish these things if the child is left entirely responsible for his own work. The consequences of leaving a worksheet on the kitchen table—which may range from missing recess to not receiving a "good job" sticker—are meaningless if the child feels that his parent is to blame for not reminding him to pack up the homework before leaving for school. A five-year-old in kindergarten will learn to return a library book if not returning it means she cannot check out another book the next day. Homework gives parents the opportunity to grant their children independence.

On the other hand, as our children grow older, it does seem necessary to keep tabs on how much time our children are spending on their homework, and to monitor the quality of the atmosphere in which they are working outside of school. Is your fourth-grader scribbling answers on a crumpled worksheet that's balanced on her lap in the car on the way to soccer practice? Is your fifth-grader bleary-eyed after staying up until one A.M. at a Saturday night sleepover, trying to build a relief map of Venezuela? Why, really, are nine-year-olds staying up until ten P.M. to cut and paste?

"I have not seen the levels of homework change over the many years I've been a school head," says a principal at a highly respected elementary school. "What's changed are the parents' perceptions of homework, and the overscheduling of children. Parents really feel they cannot not do everything. So homework takes a backseat. It's not a priority. And this will remain an issue until we have some balance in our lives again."

As we've seen, cutting back on extracurricular activities means compromising your child's formal exposure to every passing hobby or sport. Cutting back also means that there will be more time in the day for a reasonable amount of homework. What you consider reasonable is something to work out with your child and your child's school. Some children like assuming the weary, put-upon role of the homework martyr. For them, it's a matter of pride to claim that a social studies project kept them up until eleven P.M. But while it may be humbling to hear an emergency room resident plead exhaustion after working three days straight, it's only sad to see a child under twelve burning the midnight oil, and feeling righteous about it. When in doubt about home-work, communicate with teachers.

*   *   *

All of the strategies in this chapter boil down to one effort: making room in your children's lives for sleep. Many people will say to me, "Well, your kids are extraordinary. They must need a lot of sleep. Mine just don't. One's a night owl and the other is perfectly fine with eight or nine hours." Through the years I've usually just shrugged this away. But given the opportunity, I put the question to Judith Owens. What would she say to these people?

She laughed. "I wish I had a dollar for every patient who came to me and said, 'Well, my child just doesn't need that much sleep,'" Owens said. "I say to them, 'Your kid just isn't getting that much sleep. Until you prove to me otherwise, I'm going to assume that your seven-year-old, for example, needs eleven hours of sleep every night. You don't know what your kid looks like with that much sleep.' There are constitutional short-sleepers, but they are few and far between. Most parents never give kids the opportunity to get the amount they need."

After all the explanations and justifications, you finally have to ask yourself what is really keeping you from putting your children to bed early. They need the sleep; you need the time alone. Some sleep experts postulate that the problem is guilt. After a long day, working and at-home parents alike may desire nothing more than to get their kids out of the way at seven o'clock. Feeling guilty about this desire, they actually keep the children up later than is good for the children or right for the parents. Ultimately, this practice puts the whole family at risk for sleep deprivation. Generally, when the children go to bed too late, the parents, desperate for some adult time, push their own bedtime later.

"The whole process of parents relinquishing control over bedtime sets this in motion," says Judith Owens, whose work entitles her to have the last word on the subject. "Don't feel guilty for putting your kid to bed."

Food: The Life
of the Kitchen

I spend an hour in the kitchen at breakfast time, an hour or more at lunchtime, and usually two hours a day at dinnertime. That's at least four hours a day of preparing food, cooking food, serving food, eating food, and cleaning up food. I'd be interested in calculating how much more time (if any) Ma from the *Little House* books spent feeding her family more than a century ago. It's not as though I don't make use of modern conveniences; I do. I use a blender and a pressure cooker. A year ago I finally bought a Cuisinart, which expanded my repertoire considerably. I also depend upon my handheld blender, which I use for soups and purees. I admit that due to a primitivist bias I favor flames over microwaves, but that's really my only point of backwardness in the kitchen. So what's going on here? What's taking me so long?

The kitchen is our family's principle gathering place. It's the room that welcomes us as a group in the morning, and receives us when we return home. We have what realtors call an eat-in kitchen, which is very nice. It means that while I am working, my children can be with me if they'd like to. I'm not laboring in isolation. My daughter is now old enough to drift in and out of the preparation. She likes to stir pots and blend ingredients. Now that she has permission to use the stove, she likes to prepare tea for herself and her brothers. (After all these years, her recent transition from food consumer to fire-managing food preparer seems worthy of some sort of ritual observance, although I'm not sure of what sort.)

The kitchen, for me, is a place where our family feels especially familial. For this reason among many, I could not tolerate a television's blank or flashing face in this room. Even when it's off, the TV sends a message: "Hey, you might not be watching me right now, but you could be, and you might very well be missing something fun or interesting that everyone will be talking about when you get to school or work. But if you really don't want to . . ."

Radios and tape or CD players are fine.

Now it's time for the 7 o'clock bedtime meal plan, which requires a little background orientation. In general, try to avoid buying groceries that come in tons of packaging: boxes, cans, plastic tubs, and so on. Just as an early bedtime undermines and subverts those who'd like to turn your kids into rushed, fattened, harried consumers, the point of kitchen politics is to undermine the processors of bad food. There's a simple vicious cycle at play here: overworking and overscheduling create less time to prepare food, which create a demand for synthetically flavored food and instant this and that.

Just add water!

Ready after twenty-five seconds in the microwave!

Tear this open and eat it!

Such hastiness represents an asocial, atomizing way to sustain life. There's a time and a place for granola bars and squeeze yogurts. There's a time and a place for candy bars, jelly beans, and Happy Meals. But these things can't be expected to know their time and place on their own, and their manufacturers necessarily want them to find their way into our hearts.

Actually, sugar consumption plays directly into body chemistry and physiology, which in turn affects the quality of sleep. You may or may not see the effects of sugar on your child's sleep habits, but I'm sure sweets influence your life in one way or another.

Perhaps, then, this is a good moment to talk about candy. I know there has been a time in each of my children's lives when, with respect to importance, I routinely came in a plodding second to a handful of M&Ms. Frankly, I found it hard to compete against Milky Ways and gummy worms, and it was all too easy to let candy get the best of me. For one thing, it's everywhere. It's at the checkout line at the grocery store. It's used by teachers for incentive and reward. It's dumped in party favor bags. It grows and multiplies like fungi in the so-called specialty aisles around each of the major holidays. Halloween, Christmas, Hanukkah, and Valentine's Day alone create a four-month period during which children are tempted and encouraged to stuff themselves with sweets. Indeed, sugar consumption's effect on sleep regulation is itself a book topic.

A few years ago we learned of a ritual that pulled us out of our candy-induced victimhood. Our Swedish friends shared with us their Old World custom of presenting children with a bag of sweets once a week. The bag contained enough sweets to feel like a full complement of candy—enough to be savored over the course of the week—but not so much that if a child consumed all of it in once sitting he would get sick. In our family, we hide the candy bags on Sunday after lunch, and the children run around trying to find them. Midafternoon on Sunday seems to work for us because the candy doesn't ruin their appetite for dinner, nor does it seem to affect their sleep. The only catch is, they may not ask for candy any other time of the week. No begging, no whining. If they go to a birthday party and come home with a giant party favor bag filled with candy, that counts as the week's supply.

Like anything you do, Candy Day soon takes on a life of its own. I actually enjoy putting the bags together, and when interesting sweets catch my eye I include them in the next week's bags. These days you can find healthy versions of almost any kind of candy—licorice, chocolate, fruit gels, you name it—which is something to consider when planning your bags. (By healthy I mean anything edible that does not contain artificial sweeteners, colors, preservatives, genetically engineered components, or hand-me-down growth hormones.) But even I, yes, will toss in a box of Nerds from time to time, considering such a treat as a homeopathic dose of garbage.

Now let's look briefly at fats. I use butter and oil freely in my cooking. What I don't use are the faux fats: Who needs them? Either use butter and oils in moderation, or use nothing. It doesn't take a lot of imagination to envision the haunting health risks consequent to consuming these synthetic, oleaginous pastes that come packed in plastic tubs.

A working pantry really helps to keep the meals coming. Here's what you can buy in bulk and keep in your refrigerator or, in some cases, your freezer: flour, pasta, rice, oats, cold cereals, dried fruits, legumes, oils, seeds, and nuts. In the winter I also keep a case of canned plum tomatoes on hand. Once a week I buy eggs, fruits, vegetables, milk and dairy products, and the meats (if any) I plan to serve that week. Once a month I replenish my pantry. Along with the bulk items I buy corn chips, bean dip, pickles, coffee, condiments, and the other miscellaneous items. In spite of avoiding packaging whenever possible, I still find myself recycling huge loads of plastic, glass, and cardboard that accumulate each week.

The trick to staying on top of the food game is to find a rhythm that works for you. The way to find a rhythm is to work as many preparations as possible into at least two kinds of meals and/or snacks. Here's what I mean.

Say you roast a chicken on Friday night. The carcass is picked clean. When you're doing the dishes, toss the bones into a pot, cover it with a lid, and put it in the fridge. The next day, cover it with water and simmer it for a few hours. Strain the soup, add salt, and you've got chicken broth for your next meal. All you have to do is make dumplings of some kind, or cooked noodles, or steamed vegetables, and—with salad and bread—you've got another meal.

My four-year-old loves oatmeal. Cold or hot, he adores the stuff. So I leave the extra porridge in his bowl all morning and he'll eat it either as a snack or as part of lunch. I leave cold pancakes out on weekend mornings too for the same reason.

If you make a stew on a Sunday afternoon to serve for Sunday dinner, make a double portion and serve the second half on Tuesday (not Monday). I find that allowing one day between leftovers makes the meal seem a little less left over. My other rule for leftovers is that I try to introduce one new thing with each leftover meal. So if it's stew again, I'll serve it with potatoes instead of rice, or offer a dessert after the meal.

Because I am home with a preschooler between noon and three, I often prepare the evening meal after I've eaten my lunch and while my four-year-old is finishing his. This is a good time of day to prepare the things you do not have time to make during the after-school hours. If we're having chicken breasts or fish fillets, I'll mix up a marinade, pour it over the chicken or fish, and put them in the fridge. I may bake a squash, scoop out the flesh, mash it with butter, brown sugar, and cinnamon and put it aside, covered, for later reheating. I may lay out a lasagna, readying it for baking at four o'clock. I may cook black beans in the pressure cooker. I may wash the salad or the raw vegetables for a pasta sauce.

It makes sense to plan the meals around what you've got on hand. That is, use the things with the shortest shelf life first. Eat salads while the lettuce and other fixings are fresh. Toward the end of the week, make salads out of the longer-lasting items like carrots and peppers. Soups made from carrots and sweet potatoes can get you through that last day before you go grocery shopping again.

People always develop their own systems. I have working friends who have rediscovered the Crock-Pot. One woman puts her entire meal in the slow cooker right after breakfast and comes home to a hot meal at five o'clock. Another friend makes chicken stock a couple of times a month and freezes it in quartz-size batches for use all month long. Yet another woman I know cooks several meals in one evening after her children go to sleep. She freezes some, refrigerates others, and has her week's dinners preprepped.

Sometimes my four-year-old and I talk during this cooking time; other times he's off in his own world talking to himself and pretending. Sometimes he goes to his room. Sometimes he has a friend over and the two children are playing nearby. My goal, if I am preparing this way, is to be out of the kitchen by one-thirty. That leaves us an hour and a half or so of free time to spend together. Mostly we play Candyland and a highly modified Pokémon card game. I read him stories. But he is also free to go off on his own. After all, this is his only time to play freely without a big brother and sister around. He basks in totally unstructured time.

Before leaving for the afternoon carpool I assemble the car snack mentioned in chapter 2. Over the years I have experimented with all kinds of snacks. Because my seven-year-old is a vegetarian, I am forever wondering if he's getting enough protein. One day I bought a carton of protein powder and measured some of this powder into the blender with milk, banana, and a little honey. I carried the blender to the car with a couple of plastic cups. Here's my advice: Never do this. Before I pulled away from the curb the blender toppled from its resting place between my legs and spilled all over my feet and the car floor. My then three-year-old was fussing (I'd had to waken him from a nap), and my new leather clogs were in a puddle of shake. Another overreaching idea gone bust, and the car smelled for months. Now I offer protein bars that come in a wrapper.

So don't get fancy. Stick with the easy things—grapes, apples, string cheese, granola bars, bread-and-jelly sandwiches, muffins (left over from breakfast), dried fruit. If you're so inclined, quick breads are easy to prepare and make perfect snacks.

Let's say four-thirty finds you at home without having prepared anything ahead of time, even in your mind. You look in the fridge, and there's nothing but some moldy bean dip, a half gallon of milk, a couple of cheeses that nobody likes, and some rubbery celery that you haven't the heart to throw away. Look closer: maybe there are a dozen eggs you can scramble and serve with toast. Maybe you can have cold cereal. Or maybe there's a jar of prepared pasta sauce you've been keeping on hand for just such a night. When you make the effort in good faith most of the time and you fall short some of the time, your family has to accept it in good spirits. They owe you that much. Throw your hands up and say, "Oh, well!" Nobody is perfect, and chances are you are not a professional chef, whose chief characteristic is the ability to turn a pantry and refrigerator of apparent junk into a tasty meal.

It can help to plan your pizza nights ahead of time. Likewise with dinners out *en famille*. Knowing that you have a break coming up makes it easier to keep the meals coming in the press of the week.

There is nothing magical about the following collection of recipes. Most are old standbys. Simple as they are, I submit them merely as jumping-off points for your own efforts. Sometimes I will hear what somebody else is making for dinner and think to myself, "That sounds really good. Why don't I ever make anything like that?" So then I try it. Sometimes it's a hit; often it's not. And back I slink to my rut. Although I consult with cookbooks for cooking times, baking measurements, and for acquiring new ideas, I am just beginning to mess around with ingredients in what you might call an imaginative way. This is how you do it: Act like a chef. You have only the ingredients you can already find in your kitchen. Make something that tastes good.

One other thing: The following recipes may require some exegesis in order to place them into the limited context of your day and the broader context of your choices in life. Like sleep, food is not optional in life, but its quality is.

Starting the Day

GOOD MORNING OATMEAL

During the school months I make oatmeal day in and day out. Only one of my children complains that he'd sometimes like something different, so at least one or two school mornings a week I serve yogurt and granola, frozen waffles, Cream of Wheat, French toast, or cold cereal. While scratch pancakes are typically reserved for weekends, healthy versions of mixes do make pancakes an option when time is limited.

Always try to serve some kind of fresh fruit—sliced banana, grape-fruit, or berries—along with the oatmeal.

2 cups water
2 cups milk
2 cups rolled oats

Mix the water and milk in a pot. Stir in the rolled oats. Bring to a low boil and simmer ten to twelve minutes, stirring from time to time, until the mixture thickens. Turn off heat and cover for a minute or two. Serve with salt and butter, or maple syrup, or honey.

(Oatmeal variation: After stirring in the rolled oats, add one grated apple [with the peel], one tablespoon of wheat germ or flax meal, 1/2 cup of raisins, and 1/4 teaspoon of cinnamon. Continue as above.)

•*Serves three children and one adult.*

EASY PANCAKES

Just to keep myself on the up and up, I made these from scratch this morning, a cold Tuesday in February when I was under a ton of pressure to get out the door at precisely 7:30 A.M. I didn't get down to the kitchen until 6:43, but we still made it into the car by 7:39.

1 cup white flour
1 cup whole wheat flour (or spelt flour)
2 tablespoons sugar
1 1/2 teaspoons baking powder
1 teaspoon baking soda
1/8 teaspoon salt
2 tablespoons canola oil
2 eggs
1 cup plain low-fat yogurt
1 cup milk
Oil for frying

In a large bowl mix the dry ingredients. In another bowl mix the oil, eggs, yogurt, and milk. Pour wet ingredients into the dry ingredients and blend. Add milk or water to thin to desired consistency. Heat the skillet. When a drop of water skitters across the skillet it's hot enough. Spread a teaspoon or more of oil in the pan with a paper towel. Fry the pancakes and serve with real maple syrup.

(Option: Feel free to add to the batter one cup of chopped fresh fruit such as apples, bananas, or berries.)

•*Serves three children and one adult.*

SCHOOL DAY FRENCH TOAST

4 eggs
1/4 cup milk
1/4 teaspoon vanilla (optional)
Cinnamon (optional)
5 slices of stale bread
Butter or oil for frying

Beat the eggs in a casserole. Stir in milk and vanilla. Lay slices of stale (or very lightly toasted) bread in the egg mixture. When one side has absorbed the mixture, flip the slices over. Meanwhile, heat butter or oil in a skillet. When the grease is hot, spread it around the entire skillet and, lifting the soaked bread with a slotted spatula, lay the bread in the skillet. It should sizzle. Sprinkle cinnamon on the cooking bread. When the bottom is golden brown, flip the slices and cook until the egg is cooked through. Serve with maple syrup, jelly, or powdered sugar.

Hint: Cut the slices of bread in half before soaking. Then they don't fall into tatters when you lift them out of the egg.

• *Serves three children and one adult.*

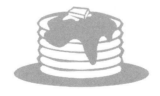

EASY BUT GOOD MUFFINS

This may be too much for most people, including me, but you really can mix up the dry ingredients the night before. Take the butter out of the fridge the night before too; then it's not too hard to smear it in the tin. (Oil is always easy to spread.) The next morning, preheat the oven when you first get downstairs, then mix up the wet ingredients, grease the muffin tin, and mix the dries and wets. While they're baking, start the oatmeal. These muffins freeze very well. When they're cool, put them in a resealable bag and set them in the freezer. Reheat in the microwave or toaster oven at 250 degrees.

1 1/2 cups whole wheat flour (or spelt flour)
1 cup wheat germ
1/2 teaspoon salt
3 teaspoons baking powder
1 cup milk (or soy milk)
1 slightly beaten egg
3 tablespoons canola oil
1/4 cup honey

Preheat oven to 400 degrees. Combine dry ingredients in a large bowl. In a separate bowl combine wet ingredients. Pour the wet into the dry and stir just until blended. Batter will be thick. Spoon into greased muffin tins and bake about twenty minutes. Serve with unsugared jelly or jam.

• *Yields about ten to twelve muffins.*

CINNAMON TOAST

Cinnamon toast is an after-school snack as well as a breakfast side dish. The fragrance and the taste of cinnamon toast makes my children feel completely good inside. I hear them boast to their friends about their mother's "famous cinnamon toast," which always reminds me how little children recognize or care for the degree of difficulty in food preparation. Indeed, when I solicited their input for this section of the book, most of the recipes they chose to pass on are so easy a child could make them. But maybe that's the point.

Three slices of bread for toasting
3 tablespoons sugar
2 teaspoons cinnamon
Butter

In a bowl mix sugar and cinnamon. Soften a stick of butter. Toast the bread. Spread with butter and sprinkle with the cinnamon mixture. Cut into triangles. Serve hot.

• *Serves three.*

Midday Cookery

The following recipes are those you might find helpful during your advance preparation time. Having them done ahead of time makes it possible to be a thirty-minute gourmet starting at four-thirty. Necessarily incomplete as this collection is, I hope it triggers ideas for things you might do that suit your own family's tastes and needs.

SALAD DRESSING I

Even a plain green salad tastes better when the dressing is homemade. Take a quart jar with a lid and mix up your salad dressing for the week. Play with the proportions as you like.

  1 shallot, peeled and quartered
  3 cloves garlic, peeled
  Salt and pepper to taste
  1 tablespoon Dijon or stone-ground mustard
  1 1/2 cups olive oil
  1 cup red wine vinegar

Mix all the ingredients in a blender. Refrigerate.

•Makes about two cups.

SALAD DRESSING II

For a while I was into creamy dressings that might pack a little protein for my vegetarian son. The idea was to pour things in the blender and see what came out.

1 tablespoon minced ginger
2 peeled garlic cloves
1/2 cup apple cider (or red wine) vinegar
2 tablespoons tamari or soy sauce
1/4 cup tahini (sesame paste)
1 tablespoon roasted sesame oil
1/4 teaspoon sugar or honey
1/4 cup canola oil

Mix all the ingredients in a blender jar. Use as a dip for raw vegetables or as a dressing. Thin if necessary with brewed tea or water. Refrigerate.

•Makes one cup.

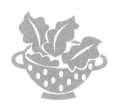

MARINADE FOR FISH, CHICKEN, AND BEEF

It took me a long time to come around to the idea of square meals. I grew up on them and consequently spent twenty years exploring the alternatives. During my years as a modified vegetarian, I became comfortable with all kinds of substitutes for the meat-starch-vegetable triumvirate. These nonexclusionary meals included beans, pasta, legumes, rice, grains, eggs, and vegetables all mixed up in any number of fanciful combinations. They were meals without borders. Now a meat eater once again, I have returned to the square meal a couple of times a week. First of all, it's often easier to prepare. Second of all, it allows people to pick and choose from the items on their plate. Everything's not all mushed up together. But a broiled chicken breast is infinitely better if you take a little time to flavor it before cooking. This is also true for that tilapia fillet or the flank steak you picked up on sale yesterday. Mix your marinade at lunchtime. Marinating reduces the cooking time, so be alert when testing for doneness.

> 2 tablespoons minced ginger
> 3 tablespoons soy sauce or tamari
> 1 teaspoon sugar
> 1/4 cup canola oil
> 1 tablespoon sesame oil
> 3 garlic cloves, minced
> 1/4 cup orange juice

Mix all the ingredients in a bowl and ladle it over the meat or fish. Keep food in the refrigerator until ready to cook.

• *Makes one cup.*

MY MOTHER'S CHAT·'N'·SLAP
MEAT LOAF

My mother prepared this recipe while talking to her friends on the phone after she got home from work. With the phone cradled between her neck and her shoulder, she'd smack the bottoms of the always near-empty condiment jars until, in spite of being utterly distracted, she had determined that just the right amount of flavor had been imparted to the mixture. It doesn't seem to matter all that much how much of any of these things you put in; this meat loaf always tastes good.

2 pounds ground beef
2 eggs, beaten
2 tablespoons water
2 tablespoons mustard
1 14-ounce jar of chili sauce
2 tablespoons matzoh meal or cracker crumbs, optional

Preheat the oven to 350 degrees. In a large bowl mix all of the ingredients. Press into a 9" x 5" loaf pan and bake for one hour. After removing from the oven, let the meat loaf stand a minute until, as my mother says, it "soaks back all the juices." Serve hot or at room temperature with mashed potatoes or rice and a tomato-and-onion salad.

•*Serves five with leftovers.*

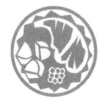

NOODLE PUDDING

Although I almost always serve this dish as a side course with brisket or roast chicken, noodle pudding can hold its own for dinner if you serve it with soup and/or a tossed salad. If you double the recipe you can always freeze one for another day.

12 ounces wide egg noodles, uncooked
2 tablespoons butter
1/4 cup sugar
1 teaspoon cinnamon
3/4 cup unsweetened applesauce
1/3 cup raisins
1/2 cup cottage cheese
4 eggs, beaten

Preheat the oven to 350 degrees. Slightly undercook the noodles according to the package directions. Drain and return to the pot. Stir in all the ingredients but the eggs. Taste for flavor and adjust as necessary. Stir in the eggs. Pour into a buttered 13" x 9" casserole and bake, covered, for 30 minutes. Remove the cover and continue baking for 30 more minutes.

•*Serves six.*

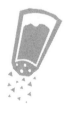

SAVORY POTATO KUGEL

he food processor may do more to bring back traditional Eastern European cookery than any number of memoirs written by emigrés who eulogize borschts and kugels. Here's why: Grating potatoes and onions by hand is a wretched enterprise. I can't stand it when my knuckles, scraped raw upon the grater, bleed into the bowl and stain the potatoes pink. It's disgusting. Also, what used to take an hour of steady grating can be done in, literally, a flash. I realize that I've spent this whole book harping upon the beauty and meaning of time, of taking the time to do things and enjoying the process by which the work of life gets done. Grating, unfortunately, is a process I detest. So when it comes to grating potatoes, carrots, apples, zucchini, cheese, and any number of other things, I'm afraid I have to side with product over process. For the sake of the variety of our menus, I do not scorn the wonder of certain high-tech blade operations.

4 eggs
8 medium russet potatoes
1 large onion, peeled and cut
6 tablespoons matzoh meal (you can substitute cracker
   crumbs)
1 1/2 teaspoons baking powder
2 teaspoons salt
1/4 teaspoon pepper
1/4 cup melted chicken fat or margarine (I substitute butter)

Preheat oven to 375 degrees. Break the eggs into a medium-sized bowl and set aside. Grate the potatoes and onion. Squeeze out the excess water and mix with the eggs. Stir in the remaining ingredients. Turn into a large, greased soufflé dish. Bake thirty to forty-five minutes until golden brown.

•*Serves six to eight.*

Soups

Soups are an obvious choice when you're looking for things to prepare ahead of time. They're also a good way of sneaking in secret ingredients like vegetables, which in plain view may elicit groans.

PAUL'S EXCELLENT DIGESTIVE SOUP

Nearly twenty years ago our friend Paul was a struggling film-maker living in Paris. He made this soup for us and told us it was good for the digestive system as long as you added no pepper. Today Paul is a physician and the digestive systems of his patients are, by all accounts, estimable.

> *3 large leeks, white part only, chopped*
> *2 tablespoons sweet butter*
> *4 carrots, diced*
> *4 medium potatoes, peeled and diced*
> *2 turnips, peeled and diced*
> *Salt to taste*
> *Fresh parsley, minced, for garnish (optional)*

Sauté the leeks in the butter. When they've turned translucent, add a splash of water and cook for a minute or two more. Add the rest of the vegetables and cover them with water. Season with salt and simmer uncovered for an hour and a half. Check for seasoning and add salt if necessary. You may serve the soup at this point. I find, however, that if I puree the soup with a handheld blender the flavors blend beautifully and the children like it better. Garnish with minced fresh parsley if desired. Serve with cheese and bread.

•*Serves six with plenty left over.*

MISO SOUP

This easy soup is made from soy bean paste, which is sold in most grocery stores and is usually kept near the vegetable section with the Asian products and the tofu. The enzymes in miso are said to be extremely nutritious; according to some, the beneficial properties of these enzymes are destroyed by excessive heat, which is why you do not simmer or boil the soup. While light, a chockful miso soup prepared with all the extras constitutes a completely balanced meal when served with rice or rice cakes. For extra protein you can always spread almond or peanut butter on the rice cakes.

1 onion, sliced
2 carrots, julienned
1 tablespoon canola oil
5 cups water
5 tablespoons brown rice miso, or to taste
Optional: chopped scallions, shredded bok choy, mung bean
    sprouts, cubed tofu (raw or sauteed), 2 tablespoons tahini
    (sesame paste) thinned with miso stock

In a large pot, sauté the chopped onion and carrots in the canola oil. Add the water and heat. In a separate bowl, blend the miso with hot water from the pot until it's thin enough to pour back into the pot. Heat through but do not simmer or boil. Before serving, add any or all of the optional ingredients.

•*Serves five.*

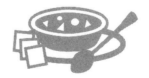

Baked Things

There's no hastening the roots, tubers, and squashes. They need time to bake, and there's nothing easier than throwing something in the oven while you're eating lunch. Potatoes of any kind can be baked, mashed, and pressed into a casserole to be reheated. Likewise for squash.

ALL·PURPOSE BEETS

Beets are packed with nutrients and are even better room temperature than hot. Trim the greens and wrap the beets individually in foil. Bake in a preheated 400-degree oven until tender. Depending on the size and age of the beets, cooking time can range from thirty minutes to about an hour. When the beets are cool, slip off their skin. Dressed with fresh dill, olive oil, and a little balsamic vinegar, they often appeal even to picky eaters.

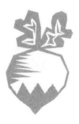

CHALLAH

On Friday afternoons I bake challah, a braided, egg-rich bread that signifies the end of the workweek and the beginning of the Jewish day of rest. The richness of the bread is analogous to the potential richness of the twenty-four hours each week during which (in theory, anyway) we cease from doing the work of the world. Whether or not I actually rest on Saturdays, baking the challah every week makes me feel good. It makes the house smell like a place I like coming home to. Further, I always know that even if the evening meal is a flop, my family will have one thing to eat that they all love. Setting up the dough takes no more than ten minutes. Also, you can halve the recipe and make one loaf instead of two.

One of my friends prepares the dough for its first rising at two o'clock so that the bread is ready for shaping when her kids come home at three-thirty. She braids one loaf—the family loaf—and divides the remaining dough into three pieces, one for each child to shape as they wish.

Recently I learned that Jews are supposed to set two challahs on the Friday night table. The double portion recollects how, recently escaped from Egypt and dependent on manna falling from the skies, the liberated slaves were required to fetch two portions of manna on Fridays, enough to last two days. On the day of rest, even the scramble for manna was suspended. Since I usually halve the recipe, occasionally I simply divide the ball into two smaller loaves. In this way I accommodate halakic rigor and simultaneously please the crust lovers. Other nights I like one big loaf. This pleases those who prefer the symbolic meaning of a plentiful and fluffy warm center.

There are many recipes for challah. This one came from a friend. She got it from her mother-in-law's sister. As we braid bread, so we braid our lives with those of our friends.

2 packages yeast
1/3 cup sugar
1 teaspoon salt
7 cups (approximately) unbleached white flour
1 1/2 cups water, very hot but not simmering
4 eggs
2/3 cup canola oil
1 cup golden raisins or currants (optional)

Combine the yeast, sugar, salt, and one cup of the flour into a large bowl. Pour the hot water into the dry ingredients and stir. Let rest for a minute or so. Stir in the eggs, oil, and four cups flour. Continue to add flour until you have a kneadable ball. (Usually about two more cups.) Add one cup of golden raisins if desired. Knead for two or three minutes. Cover and place in a dark corner (I use the cold oven) for an hour and a half to let the dough rise. Punch down, knead a little more, and divide the large ball into two balls.

Divide one of the balls into four equal pieces. Squeeze and stretch the pieces into snakes and lay them parallel on a greased baking sheet. Tweak them together at the center. Braid from the center to the ends on one side, then repeat on the other side. Brush with beaten egg. Repeat for the other loaf. Place the braided loaves in a dark corner and let rise a half hour more. Preheat oven to 350 degrees and bake for twenty-five to thirty minutes.

•*Makes 2 large loaves.*

Quick Breads

One other thing I may do at lunchtime is bake a quick bread for snacks. You can divide the dough into muffin tins lined with paper, or make a single loaf. If I don't mind wrestling with a large amount of batter, I'll make enough for two loaves and freeze one. I've adapted the first recipe from the muffins my son's class prepared and served on Mother's Day. The second comes from *Jane Brody's Good Food Book*. Incidentally, I consider quick breads made with carrot and zucchini to be vegetables.

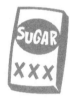

BLUE ROOM BANANA BREAD

1 cup butter (you may substitute canola oil)
2 cups sugar
3 eggs
2$\frac{1}{2}$ cups mashed banana
$\frac{3}{4}$ to 1 cup plain low-fat yogurt
4$\frac{1}{8}$ cups flour (I use half whole wheat, half white)
1$\frac{1}{2}$ teaspoons baking powder
1$\frac{1}{2}$ teaspoons baking soda
$\frac{3}{4}$ teaspoon salt
Optional: raisins, chocolate chips, chopped dates

Preheat the oven to 350 degrees. In a large bowl, cream the butter and sugar. Add the eggs, banana, and yogurt and mix well. In a separate bowl, mix the dry ingredients. Blend the wet and dry ingredients, adding more yogurt if the batter seems too dry. Stir in a handful of any of the optional ingredients, if desired. Turn into two buttered loaf pans. Bake about forty-five minutes, or until a toothpick inserted in the center comes out clean.

Hint: If you substitute canola oil for the butter, treat it as a wet ingredient and blend the oil with the eggs and banana.

•Makes two loaves.

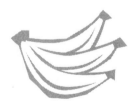

APPLESAUCE·CARROT CAKE

1 1/2 cups white flour
1/2 cup whole wheat flour
2/3 cup sugar
2 teaspoons baking soda
1 1/2 teaspoons cinnamon
1/2 teaspoon nutmeg
1/2 teaspoon salt, if desired
3/4 cup applesauce
1/4 cup oil
3 large eggs, or 2 egg whites and 2 whole eggs
3 cups coarsely grated carrots

Preheat the oven to 350 degrees. In a large bowl, combine the dry ingredients. In a separate bowl, combine everything else except the carrots. Mix the wet ingredients into the dry ingredients. Add the carrots, and mix again. Pour the batter into a greased 9" tube pan. Bake about one hour ten minutes or until a toothpick inserted in the thickest part of the cake comes out clean. Set the cake on a wire rack to cool for five minutes. Run a knife around the edges of the pan to loosen the cake, and turn the cake out onto the wire rack to cool.

•Makes one cake.

Salads and Side Dishes

Children smile when you put something on their plate that is pretty or inventive. My sons think cream cheese toast is one of the seven wonders of the world because I cut it into an elephant head before setting it before them. Once the bread is toasted and spread with cream cheese, I cut a triangle out of the center of the toast, using the bottom edge of the toast as the base. Then I slide the triangle point-side upward and the two remaining exterior wedges downward until the triangle looks like a trunk and the wedges like big ears, only upside down. I may put a couple of raisins on either side of the trunk for eyes. Make sure you orient the plate so that the face is facing your child.

When my seven-year-old was in preschool, he (like many kids) liked to come home to the exact same lunch every single day: elephant cream cheese toast and a bowl of lemon yogurt. Around the top half of the yogurt I would spoon a fringe of hair, actually wheat germ. Raisins formed eyes, nose, and mouth. Eventually I would make eyebrows out of red pepper slivers (which I might be slicing for the evening salad). Back in the hard old days with a napping toddler, a four-year-old, and a kindergartner, I'd get back from the noon carpool and have to dash the toddler off to bed so that he could get in a two-hour nap before the afternoon pickup at three. My middle child quite often ate his lunch alone, listening to music while I put the toddler down for his nap. Then I'd come back down and proceed with lunch cleanup and dinner prep as detailed above.

And way, way back in the really, really hard old days, I used to prepare many a meal with an infant or toddler in the backpack. Now that I think about it, when our third child was between six and eighteen months old, he usually was fed and put to bed by six. I can see him now in his high chair fingering bits of cheese toast and raisins as I prepared the regular meal. I think my husband would get home from work and finish off the dinner prep while I'd put the baby to bed. Then we'd have dinner with the three- and five-year-olds. Somehow they'd still get to bed by seven.

This is a long digression from my point that the appearance of food on the plate really matters to young children, and it's not something to discourage. Now that the children are older, I expect them to eat the things that they must eat without too much complaint and without little decorative devices helping them along. And in fact, our kids have fairly well-rounded appetites and the will to try most things at least once. Still, I do try to make food look appetizing and taste good, if only because it teaches them to bring an artistic, critical sensibility to everything they do in life, and not only to the limited range of activities that people call art.

COLORFUL CARROT AND APPLE SLAW

4 carrots, scraped and trimmed at the ends
1 apple, washed and cored

Grate the carrots and apple in a food processor. Toss the apple-carrot mixture in a bowl with a little honey and lemon juice.

Hint: **You might add minced celery for extra crunch.**

•*Serves five as a side dish.*

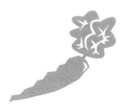

RED SALAD

2 beets, baked, peeled, and cut into walnut-size cubes
1/2 cup walnut pieces
1/4 cup scallions, chopped
2 Granny Smith apples, cored and cubed as above
Cold-pressed, extra virgin olive oil to taste
Red wine vinegar to taste

Toss all the ingredients together and dress with oil and vinegar or Salad Dressing I on page 140. Serve with a chunk of goat cheese (chevre), blue cheese, or feta on a bed of lettuce.

•Serves five.

Variations on Broccoli

I think we can all agree that broccoli is good for you. Try to get it in at least once or twice a week.

A friend serves broccoli to her family almost every night of the week. She steams the florets and then places them under the broiler with a little cheddar cheese on top. When the cheese is melted, it's ready.

My sister serves a dish she calls jungle broccoli. She steams the stalks and balances them like trees on the plate so that they stand upright like a miniature forest. Her children pretend to be dinosaurs nibbling vegetation during the Jurassic period.

Last summer my sister made a pasta sauce out of leftover broccoli and a few stubs of old blue cheese. In a saucepan she melted butter, then added the cheese and a little milk. She stirred in a spoonful of flour and cooked the sauce until it thickened, stirring constantly. She added salt and pepper and tossed the sauce with cooked penne. It was delicious. For some reason even those inimical to broccoli seem to like it when it's made with some sort of cheese.

One of my favorite broccoli dishes sounds like nothing special but somehow tastes great.

BROCCOLI MAC

1 generous tablespoon olive oil
1 garlic clove, minced
4 cups water
2 tablespoons tomato paste
1 teaspoon salt
Pepper to taste
4 cups chopped broccoli
1 cup whole wheat (or regular) shells or macaroni
Grated Parmesan cheese

Heat the oil in a three-quart pot and sauté the garlic until lightly golden. Add the water, tomato paste, salt, and pepper to taste. Bring to a boil. Add the broccoli. Cover and simmer for five minutes. Add the pasta, cover, and simmer ten more minutes, or until tender. Sprinkle with lots of cheese and serve.

•Serves five.

CREAM OF BROCCOLI SOUP

1 onion, chopped
2 heads broccoli, chopped (about 7 cups)
1 tablespoon olive oil
4 garlic cloves, minced
2 cups low-fat milk
3 cups water
2 tablespoons whole wheat flour
2 tablespoons cornstarch
Salt to taste
Grated Parmesan or cheddar cheese to taste

Steam the broccoli until tender. In a soup pot, heat oil and saute the garlic and onion until soft. Add the steamed broccoli, milk, and water. Puree with handheld blender. While stirring, add the whole wheat flour and the cornstarch. Keep stirring and heat through until the soup thickens. Salt to taste. Serve hot with grated Parmesan or cheddar cheese.

•Serves six generously.

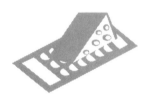

Pasta

My paternal grandparents used to buy tuna by the case. For lunch they ate tuna salad just about every day of the week. Even now, when my ninety-year-old grandmother visits I always serve a tuna salad with a side of raw scallions. Chowing down heartily, she says, "What would we do without tuna?"

Me, I'd have to pose the same question, only regarding pasta. What would we do without it? If I permitted it, my seven-year-old would eat penne with vinegar and salt every single night. If I'm feeling particularly open-minded, and if he's eaten his portion of salad or vegetable, I'll even allow him to add both cider and balsamic vinegars to his pasta. I figure by the time he graduates from high school he ought to be thoroughly pickled.

If four-thirty finds you utterly uninspired, you can always make pasta. Open a can of plum tomatoes, heat them up, and pour them over the pasta. If you like garlic, sauté several minced cloves in a generous amount of olive oil and add minced parsley. Serve this plain over cooked pasta. If summer is lingering and you have basil and tomatoes hanging around, you can make Evelyn's Cold Chop.

EVELYN'S COLD CHOP

1 pound spaghetti (penne, linguini, rotini, or any other pasta)
4 cloves garlic, minced
2 cups chopped fresh tomatoes (about 6 to 8 plum tomatoes
   or 3 beefsteak tomatoes)
1 packed cup of fresh basil, coarsely chopped
1/4 cup or more cold-pressed extra virgin olive oil
Salt to taste
Freshly ground black pepper to taste
Grated Romano cheese (optional)

Prepare the pasta and drain. Toss the rest of the ingredients into the steaming noodles. Season with salt and pepper. Garnish with grated Romano cheese if desired. You may substitute arugula for the basil.

•Serves four or five.

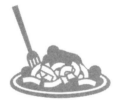

TOM'S PASTA

. . . .

The following dish is a family favorite. It's been our daughter's birthday dinner more than twice.

> 5 cloves garlic, minced
> 1/4 cup extra virgin olive oil
> 1 28-ounce can plum tomatoes
> 1 pound spaghetti
> 1 2-ounce tin anchovy fillets, minced
> 1/3 cup toasted pine nuts
> 1/3 cup capers
> 3/4 cup pitted Kalamata olives
> 1 large bunch Italian, flat leaf parsley, chopped fairly fine
> Grated Parmesan or Romano cheese (optional)

While the water is coming to a boil, prepare the ingredients for the sauce. Sauté the garlic in the olive oil. Before the garlic browns, add the can of plum tomatoes, liquid and all. Simmer the tomatoes until some of the liquid cooks off. While the tomatoes are simmering, cook the pasta.

To the reduced tomatoes add the minced anchovies and stir until the fish is dissolved. Just before the pasta is ready to be drained, mix into the sauce the toasted pine nuts, capers, and the olives. Drain the pasta, then add the parsley to the sauce. The sauce should be very green and thick. Toss the sauce with the pasta and garnish with grated Romano or Parmesan cheese.

•Serves four.

KIDS' FAVORITE TOMATO SOUP

When she was in second grade, my daughter told her teachers about the delicious tomato soup her mother made. Her teachers asked her to bring in the recipe. Here it is:

Take one 28-ounce can of Millina's Organic Plum Tomatoes. Open it. Pour the contents into a saucepan. Heat through. Blend with handheld blender. Serve piping hot.

•*Serves three children.*

BLACK BEANS AND RICE

With a pressure cooker, this meal takes forty-five minutes to prepare, but it's always worth it. The beans can be made midday.

For the beans
2 cups black turtle beans, picked over and rinsed
3 tablespoons olive oil
8 cups water
Red wine (left over from an opened bottle is ideal) or beer to taste
Blackstrap molasses to taste
Fresh lemon juice to taste
Salt to taste
Cumin to taste (optional)

For the rice
4 cups water
2 cups brown rice, rinsed well

For the topping
2 sweet red peppers, chopped
1 onion, chopped
4 cloves garlic, minced
$1/4$ cup olive oil
1 cup parsley, chopped

For the garnish:
Cheddar cheese, grated
Extra parsley, chopped
Lemon wedges
Corn chips
Tabasco sauce

Beans

Combine the beans, oil, and water in the pressure cooker. Bring the cooker to a rock and cook for thirty-five minutes. While the beans are cooking, prepare the rice. Remove the beans from the heat and cool the lid under running cold water.

Rice

Bring 4 cups water to a boil in a saucepan. Stir in the rice. Reduce the heat and let simmer uncovered about a half hour. When most of the water is absorbed and the grains are tender, turn off the heat, cover, and let rest until serving.

Topping

While the rice and beans are cooking, chop the vegetables. Sauté the onion and garlic in the olive oil. Add the peppers and cook until tender. Stir in the parsley. Keep warm.

When the beans are fully cooked, they should be tender and mashable. Mash them with a fork or potato masher or puree them with a handheld blender. Add red wine or beer, blackstrap molasses, lemon juice, salt, and cumin to taste. Blend thoroughly. Keep the beans hot, stirring to make sure they don't stick to the bottom of the pressure cooker.

To serve, scoop a portion of rice on each plate, then layer on the beans, the toppings, and the cheese. Garnish with extra parsley, lemon wedges, and corn chips. Put a bottle of Tabasco on the table for those who like their beans to have a kick.

•*Serves five with plenty of leftovers.*

MY SISTER'S BROWNIES:
THE ALL·TIME BEST DESSERT

L ast night I served dessert—brownies and an assortment of ice creams for the whole family. The table fell silent as we savored each spoonful. Sweets at the right time cast a spell over young and old alike, and nothing is as magical as brownies and ice cream.

These ambrosial hunks were the talk of West Berlin in the heady days before the wall came down, when my sister marketed them through neighborhood cafés. Serve them under two scoops of coffee Häagen-Dazs to those who know what freedom means, and even to those who don't.

2 sticks (1 cup) sweet butter
1 cup good-quality Dutch-processed cocoa powder
4 eggs
2 cups sugar
1 cup flour
Pinch of salt

Preheat the oven to 350 degrees. Melt the butter in a saucepan. Stir in the cocoa and let cool to room tempera-ture. With an electric mixer, or by hand, blend the eggs and sugar in a large bowl until the mixture turns pale yellow and makes a ribbon when you hoist a spoonful and let it fall back into the bowl. Stir the chocolate/butter mixture into the egg mixture. Stir in the flour and the pinch of salt. Pour into a well-buttered 9" square pan and bake until just barely set. Begin checking the pan after fifteen minutes. Do not over-bake. Let cool and slice into squares. The brownies freeze best if you don't slice them first. Feel free to halve or double the recipe.

•*Makes 20 brownies.*

Bibliography: Books to Live By

I read, therefore I am; I am, therefore I read. Both statements are true for me. For this reason it would be preposterous to suggest that only a certain number of books influenced the writing of this one. Every piece of fiction and nonfiction, every magazine article, every *label* I've ever read, has shaped me into the person I am. Still, the purpose of the following two-part annotated bibliography is to provide you with a limited number of sources that will support, either theoretically or practically, the establishment of the 7 o'clock bedtime. Instinct and observant common sense will carry you far within the confines of your family, but when people begin to question what you're up to, it's nice to know which volumes to wave around.

The first list is short. I have deliberately kept the should-have list brief because, in this instance anyway, quality is certainly more important than quantity. Finding a few books that really serve the subject is more important than filling up your nightstand with ancillary studies and polemics you'll never read.

The second list is a bit longer and reflects the books that specifically address some of the issues covered in this book. If you find any of the sources listed below especially illuminating, you can always check bibliographies and proceed with some research of your own.

THE SHOULD-HAVES

Weissbluth, Marc, M.D. *Healthy Sleep Habits, Happy Child: A Step-by-Step Program for a Good Night's Sleep.* New York: Ballantine, 1999.

If you have only one book about children and sleep, make it this one. Weissbluth uses science, scholarship, experience, and sympathy to develop step-by-step ways of establishing good sleep for children of all ages (which means good sleep for yourself). The principal revelation of the book—that children fall asleep more easily when they are not too tired—made the scales fall from my eyes. In addition to providing patterns and rhythms that you can follow in order to prevent problems from arising, Weissbluth offers cures for problems that you may have with older children. He places the human need for good sound sleep in its rightfully preeminent place beside food and shelter, which in turn solidifies your resolve when you're plagued by guilt and worry.

Dement, William C., M.D., Ph.D. *The Promise of Sleep.* New York: Delacorte, 1999.

Considered by many sleep authorities to be the grandfather of sleep medicine, Dr. Dement has pulled together in one volume a historical overview of human investigations into sleep, a harrowing look at the cost of sleep deprivation among adults, a description of current methodologies for treating sleep disorders, and a self-help section for use by the average reader. If the benefits of early bedtimes for children are still in doubt, this book makes a very good case for setting up proper sleep hygiene before bad habits and cultural pressure weigh in during the teenage years and later.

Baldwin Dancy, Rahima. *You Are Your Child's First Teacher.* Berkeley, California: Celestial Arts, 1989.

I read this book over and over again before my first child was born, and for months into her infancy. I hadn't looked at it in ten years before returning to it for the sake of this book. As I reread sections that I had thumbed over dozens of times, I was flabbergasted at how much of its sense, orientation, and suggestions I have retained, and how certain practices Baldwin Dancy mentions I had come to believe originated in my own family.

If you are familiar with the principles developed by educator and philosopher Rudolf Steiner, you will feel right at home in these pages. Baldwin Dancy provides overviews of child development, as well as suggestions for age-appropriate activities that nurture the various modes of learning in a growing human—musical, artistic, linguistic, physical, and social, among others. She emphasizes the importance of play and fantasy in fully realizing any of these modes.

Particularly germane to the 7 o'clock bedtime is chapter 11, "Rhythm and Discipline in Home Life."

Faber, Adele, and Elaine Mazlish. *How to Talk So Kids Will Listen & Listen So Kids Will Talk.* New York: Avon Books, 1980.

It says on the cover that more than two million copies of this book have been sold, so I imagine that most of you have it already. In case you don't, the authors are both disciples of the late child psychologist Dr. Haim Ginott and ardent advocates for methods of communicating that, as they write, "affirm the dignity and humanity of both parents and children."

Using real-life examples, illustrative cartoons, and open-ended exercises that you can do at home, the book provides positive strategies for establishing open and healthy communication between you and your child. It's often very hard to know what to say. We are so afraid of saying the wrong thing, and changing something so central as bedtime seems like an open invitation to battle. I strongly advise you to read *How to Talk* before launching into a new way of life.

Fuchs-Kreimer, Rabbi Nancy. *Parenting as a Spiritual Journey: Deepening Ordinary and Extraordinary Events into Sacred Occasions.* Woodstock, Vermont: Jewish Lights, 1996.

Fuchs-Kreimer braids her own contemporary, working-mother insights with mythic, folkloric, and religious traditions and a vast amount of parental anecdote in order to rewrite the everydayness of life into what might be termed spiritual italics. Though we easily forget to do so, it is possible to move through the day on two planes simultaneously—the sacred and the profane. The stories Fuchs-Kreimer tells and the collection of stories she has recorded affirm the importance of parenting on both levels, and show a reader how it can be done. Moving hour by hour through the parenting day, she demonstrates how we can establish and allow passage between the planes, with the hope of eventually commuting back and forth as freely as the angels on Jacob's ladder.

Zand, Janet, Rachel Walton, and Bob Rountree. *Smart Medicine for a Healthier Child.* New York: Avery, 1994.

When one of our children falls ill, this is the book I pick up. The three authors have compiled a comprehensive, alphabetically ordered guide to the various illnesses and ailments that befall children. For each problem they describe in detail the range of alternatives for treatment: conventional, herbal, homeopathic, flower remedies, acupressure, and diet and nutrition. For a person like me who tends to dabble in each of these systems, having them all laid out in one source eases the anxiety I experience when I fear I'm neglecting some possible remedy.

The book gives a brief description of each of the treatment modes and provides a number of useful charts and guidelines for the various medications. Specific instructions on the recommended therapies and procedures are also included. Since acquiring *Smart Medicine* I have not used any other medical reference.

Rombauer, Irma S., and Marion Rombauer Becker. *The Joy of Cooking.* New York: Bobbs-Merrill, 1975.

Because I'm limiting myself to citing only one should-have cookbook, it's got to be this one. My copy of *Joy*, which a college friend gave me in 1979, is battered and stained. Certain pages when opened release clouds of white flour. Whole sections have separated from the spine. Still, I consult it the way you'd consult a well-meaning and well-respected parent: I read the recipes with an open but independent mind and sometimes follow exactly what they suggest, particularly when baking cakes. More often than not I tinker with the amounts and ingredients in order to produce what I'm aiming for. While I would be very sad if a fire consumed all of my other cookbooks, some of which hold some of my favorite recipes, I would feel utterly at sea without *The Joy of Cooking*. It's the compass of my kitchen.

Bennett, Steve, and Ruth Bennett. *365 TV-Free Activities You Can Do with Your Child.* Holbrook, Massachusetts: Bob Adams, 1991.

This chunky, homespun little book is full of ideas that are worth trying out. Some artsy activities, like making your own sewing cards with a hole puncher and cardboard, were instant hits in our house. Other suggestions require only your time and are even better. In "What's Different About Me?" one of the players (parent or child) allows the other player(s) to have a good look at him Then he walks out of the room and returns with some small modification in his appearance. Maybe he took off a sock. Maybe he combed his hair to the other side. The ideas are great, but the best thing about this book (and others like it) is the implicit message it sends when you happen to see it on your bookshelf: Turn off the TV and do something else.

For Extra Support

Bettelheim, Bruno. *The Uses of Enchantment: The Meaning and Importance of Fairy Tales*. New York: Alfred A. Knopf, 1976.

I know, I know. The late Bettelheim had a few skeletons in his closet that popped out some years back and tarnished his reputation. Still, I admire this book, if for no other reason than because it presents a way of thinking about something we might otherwise take for granted.

Brody, Jane E. *Jane Brody's Good Food Book: Living the High-Carbohydrate Way*. New York: Bantam, 1985.

This cookbook is a valuable resource for those absolutely in the dark about stocking a kitchen and planning menus. Many of the recipes have weathered the years just fine. I do make allowances, however, for Brody's mid-1980s obsession with fat and salt, and doctor my versions of her recipes accordingly. The faux fried chicken legs on page 421 are delicious and easy.

Curran, Dolores. *Traits of a Healthy Family: Fifteen Traits Commonly Found in Healthy Families by Those Who Work with Them*. Minneapolis, Minnesota: Winston Press, 1983.

This book jumped off the library shelf into my hands simply because of its title. It's a feel-good kind of book (Curran admits that no family could come close to exhibiting all of these traits at one time) and definitely seems a little biased in favor of organized religion. But the author did survey representatives from a range of people who work directly with families in education, health, the church, family counseling, and volunteering activities. Curran lists the fifteen traits as follows: "The healthy family communicates and listens; affirms and supports one another; teaches respect for others; develops a sense of trust; has a sense of play and humor; exhibits a sense of shared responsibility; teaches a sense of right and wrong; has a strong sense of family in which rituals and traditions abound; has a balance of interaction among members; has a shared religious core; respects the privacy of one another; values service to others; fosters family table time and conversation; shares leisure time; admits to and seeks help with problems."

Elkind, David. *The Hurried Child: Growing Up Too Fast Too Soon.* New York: Addison-Wesley, 1988.

When you find yourself quitting Cub Scouts, tee ball, and third-grade band, pick up this book to make yourself feel better. "A philosophy of life, an art of living, is essentially a way of decentering," Elkind writes, "a way of looking at our lives in perspective and of recognizing the needs and rights of others. If we can overcome some of the stresses of our adult lives and decenter, we can begin to appreciate the value of childhood with its own special joys, sorrows, worries, and rewards. Valuing childhood does not mean seeing it as a happy innocent period but, rather, as an important period of life to which children are entitled."

Ferber, Richard, M.D. *Solve Your Child's Sleep Problems.* New York: Simon & Schuster, 1985.

Back in 1990, I read this book out of desperation. I pored over it like a holy text, memorizing the hours and sleep patterns of Ferber's various subjects—schedule-less Jimmy, overhydrated Sandy, early-rising Nina—until the times and cures set my sleep-deprived head spinning. As I wrote earlier, our daughter did not entirely oblige us by allowing herself to become Ferberized, but our attempt to straighten out her sleep certainly began with this book. If nothing else, I learned what she needed from her sleep, and how to track her sleep patterns with the chart Ferber provides on page 105. Ideally, Ferber's anecdotal and scientific evidence combined with Weissbluth's practical approach and method form a strategy for handling children's sleep that I heartily endorse. Also, Appendix A offers a helpful list of appropriate, bedtime/ sleep-related stories for children.

Goldbeck, Nikki, and David Goldbeck. *American Wholefoods Cuisine.* New York: Ceres Press, 1983.

This cookbook is really the *Joy of Cooking* for the vegetarian set. For the uninitiated, the authors provide extensive information about the ingredients they use and suggestions for stocking a whole-foods pantry. The section on short-order meals is particularly helpful when you draw a blank at four-thirty and need to put something on the table by five.

Condiments, casseroles, quick breads, savory pies: This book is filled with things that you can prepare early in the day or over the weekend for freezing.

Griffith, Mary. *The Homeschooling Handbook,* revised second edition. Rocklin, California: Prima, 1999.

It's nice to have this book on hand, partly to remind you of what you're not doing, and partly to give you a glimpse of a way out of the rat race. Of course, many of the ideas and suggestions for activities and approaches can be applied to the hours you have with your child after school and on weekends.

Healy, Jane M., Ph.D. *Endangered Minds: Why Children Don't Think— and What We Can Do About It.* New York: Simon & Schuster, 1990.

Here's one of those books you can point to when your friends tell you that you are overinvested in the day-to-day routine and welfare of your kids. A brain scientist, Healy discusses the overwhelming cultural changes that are producing a certain kind of human being who displays a certain constellation of alarming symptoms. She takes on TV and video, child care, and a host of other hot-button topics. Healy has an ax to grind for sure, but the information she shapes into her whetstone is compelling and, to me, persuasive.

————. *Failure to Connect: How Computers Affect Our Children's Minds—and What We Can Do About It.* New York: Simon & Schuster, 1999.

This is a book for your right hand while your left is thumbing through *Endangered Minds.* Healy is no Luddite; she acknowledges that she was predisposed to see the better side of technology when applied to children. Still, her research and conclusions may shock parents who really think that prepubescent children suffer no ill effects from unlimited screen time. She describes the symptoms of computer addiction and suggests ways to detox your child.

OTHER SOURCES CONSULTED

Berry, Mary Frances. *The Politics of Parenthood: Childcare, Women's Rights, and the Myth of the Good Mother.* New York: Viking Penguin, 1993.

Brooks, Andrée Aelion. *Children of Fast-Track Parents: Raising Self-Sufficient and Confident Children in an Achievement-Oriented World.* New York: Viking, 1989.

Carskadon, Mary A. "When Worlds Collide: Adolescent Need for Sleep Versus Societal Demands." *Phi Delta Kappan,* January 1999, p. 348.

Crispin Miller, Mark. *Boxed In: The Culture of TV.* Evanston, Illinois: Northwestern University Press, 1988.

Eliade, Mircea. *The Sacred and the Profane: The Nature of Religion: The Significance of Religious Myth, Symbolism, and Ritual Within Life and Culture.* New York: Harcourt Brace Jovanovich, 1957.

Faludi, Susan. *Backlash: The Undeclared War Against American Women.* New York: Doubleday, 1991.

Ginott, Dr. Haim G. *Between Parent and Child: New Solutions to Old Problems.* New York: The Macmillan Company, 1965.

Hewlett, Sylvia Ann. *When the Bough Breaks: The Cost of Neglecting Our Children.* New York: HarperCollins, 1991.

Hymowitz, Kay S. *Ready or Not: Why Treating Children as Small Adults Endangers Their Future—and Ours.* New York: The Free Press, 1999.

Kohn, Alfie. *Punished by Rewards: The Trouble with Gold Stars, Incentive Plans, A's, Praise, and Other Bribes.* New York: Houghton Mifflin, 1993.

Winn, Marie. *Children Without Childhood: Growing Up Too Fast in the World of Sex and Drugs.* New York: Pantheon, 1984.

Wolfson, Amy R., and Mary A. Carskadon. "Sleep Schedules and Daytime Functioning in Adolescents." *Child Development* 69, no. 4 (August 1998): 875.

Youcha, Geraldine. *Minding the Children: Childcare in America from Colonial Times to the Present.* New York: Scribner, 1995.

Acknowledgments

I thank Jay Podhoretz, who observed my life and said, "There's your book." The seven o'clock bedtime is my idea; *The 7 O'clock Bedtime* was entirely his.

I thank Cassie Jones, my editor at ReganBooks, for her great skill and good cheer. At ReganBooks I also thank Judith Regan, Shannon Ceci, Kelli Bagley, Ron de la Peña, Pam Pfeifer, Carl Raymond, Lucy Albanese, and Kurt Andrews.

I thank the many parents and children who freely shared with me the stories of their bedtimes.

INDEX